**PEDIATRIC NURSE PRACTITIONER
CERTIFICATION REVIEW**

PEDIATRIC NURSE PRACTITIONER CERTIFICATION REVIEW

Edited by

Terry E. Tippett Neilson, R.N., M.S.N.

Donna M. Behler, R.N., M.S.N.
Assistant Professors
School of Nursing
Vanderbilt University
Nashville, Tennessee

A Wiley Medical Publication
JOHN WILEY & SONS
New York • Chichester • Brisbane • Toronto • Singapore

Cover design: Wanda Lubelska
Production Editor: Cheryl Howell

Library of Congress Cataloging in Publication Data:

Pediatric nurse practitioner.

  "A Wiley medical publication."
  Includes index.
  1. Pediatric nursing. 2. Pediatric nursing—
Examinations, questions, etc. 3. Nurse practitioners.
I. Tippett Neilson, Terry Ellen. II. Behler, Donna M.
RJ245.P39   1983   610.73'62'076   82-20054
ISBN 0-471-86411-0

Printed in the United States of America

10 9 8 7 6 5 4 3 2 1

In memory of Alexander Hugh Neilson
whose life of song inspired us to go on.

CONTRIBUTORS

Donna M. Behler, R.N,, M.S.N.
Assistant Professor
School of Nursing
Vanderbilt University
Nashville, Tennessee

Beverly Bitterman, R.N., C., M.S.N.
Family Nurse Clinician
Fairview Community Health Clinic
Fairview, Tennessee

Jamie S. Brodie, R.N., C., M.S.N.
Adjunct Instructor
School of Nursing
Vanderbilt University
Director of Health Services
Tennessee Department of Corrections
Nashville, Tennessee

Pamela K. Busher, R.N., C., M.S.N.
Family Nurse Clinician
Cheatham County Health Care Center
Ashland City, Tennessee

Shirley B. Caldwell, R.N., C., M.S.N.
Family Nurse Clinician
Vanderbilt University Occupational Health Services
Assistant Professor
Community Health Nursing
School of Nursing
Vanderbilt University
Nashville, Tennessee

Lucinda L. Carlson, R.N., C., M.S.N.
Family Nurse Clinician
Metropolitan Health Department
Nashville, Tennessee

Judith Leavitt Devlin, R.N., M.S., A.N.P.
Family Nurse Clinician
Vanderbilt University Student Health Services
Formerly Nurse Clinician
Pediatric Cardiology
Vanderbilt University Medical Center
Nashville, Tennessee

John W. Greene, M.D.
Director, Division of Adolescent Medicine
Vanderbilt University
Nashville, Tennessee

Rosalie Hammond Pazulinec, R.N., C., M.S.N.
Pediatric Nurse Practitioner
Harvard University Health Service
Cambridge, Massachusetts

Cindy S. Selleck, R.N., C., M.S.N.
Assistant Professor
University of Alabama in Birmingham
Birmingham, Alabama

Martha Hudson Snow, R.N., C., M.S.N.
Family Nurse Clinician
Maternal–Infant Care Clinic
Metropolitan General Hospital
Nashville, Tennessee

Terry E. Tippett Neilson, R.N., M.S.N.
Assistant Professor
School of Nursing
Vanderbilt University
Nashville, Tennessee

Anne L. Turner, R.N., M.N.
Clinical Nurse Specialist
Diabetes Research and Training Center
Vanderbilt University
Adjunct Instructor
Community Health Nursing
School of Nursing
Vanderbilt University
Nashville, Tennessee

PREFACE

Nurse practitioners provide health care to people and families of all ages in many settings. Their preparation for practice ranges from continuing education to graduate level programs. With such diversity, mechanisms to assure high quality client care are necessary. The certification by a professional organization is one such avenue.

This book is one of two volumes designed to help the nurse practitioner and nurse practitioner student learn about children's health care. The primary intent of the book is to serve as a review for related American Nurses' Association (ANA) certification exams. As such, it can be used in self-study endeavors as well as group-initiated study. The editors recommend the use of a standard physical assessment text during the review process. In addition, it will augment resources used in formal adult, pediatric, and family nurse practitioner programs.

The format is deliberately simple. Each volume is divided into chapters that approximate the subject areas in the ANA Certification Test Content Outline. Each chapter includes specific primary health care problems (content areas) followed by study questions and a bibliography or a reference list. Each content area contains a succinct review of relevant pathophysiology, nursing assessment, and management of those problems.

As coeditors, we share with the reader our appreciation for the nurse practitioner's role. We recognize the need for peer support and encouragement as we continue to define our scope of practice.

Terry E. Tippett Neilson
Donna M. Behler

CONTENTS

PEDIATRIC NURSE PRACTITIONER CERTIFICATION REVIEW

CHAPTER 1

ISSUES IN PRIMARY HEALTH CARE

Jamie S. Brodie

Issues in primary health care encompass a variety of topics with regard to health behaviors of patients and the delivery of optimal patient care in an efficient, cost-effective manner. Selected relevant issues will be discussed in this chapter. These include the health belief model, quality assurance, regional health planning, the Professional Standards Review Organization (PSRO), and problem-oriented records.

THE HEALTH BELIEF MODEL

Modifying human behavior and particularly health-related behavior is a little-understood phenonemon. We have little knowledge about the real motivations of persons with good health habits versus those exhibiting behaviors associated with poor health. Often, despite the best health teaching, recommendations, or personal intentions, the result may be health behaviors that are neither logical nor anticipated. This can lead only to the assumption that the dynamics of health-related behavior are indeed complex. The *health belief model* is a theoretical framework with which to understand such dynamics better. Nurse practitioners are involved in the care of clients with medical problems, for whom compliance behavior or modification of behavior is an integral part of their treatment programs, for example, diabetes, hypertension, weight reduction, or nonsmoking programs. Therefore, the nurse practitioner can benefit from examining the relationship between health beliefs and human behavior.

The health belief model originated from early public health research on factors influencing compliance with preventive health measures. A basic

1

premise of the model is that health-related behavior is largely a function of the person's beliefs and perceptions. It is useful in explaining human motivation, health-seeking behavior, illness behavior, and sick-role behavior, and has clinical importance as a tool for understanding the relationship between health beliefs and the likelihood of compliance with a recommended health action. Knowledge of the motivational forces underpinning health-related behaviors can assist the nurse practitioner in the selection of the nursing intervention(s) most likely to positively influence the client's health-related behavior.

Figure 1 illustrates the components of the model and the many factors that influence individual perceptions and the likelihood of action. According to the health belief model, the likelihood of a person's engaging in a health-influencing activity involves a complex value judgment, based on the perceived threat of the condition or disease, the perceived benefits of the action, and the perceived barriers to action. The existence of modifying factors can heighten or diminish the perception of susceptibility, seriousness, or threat of a disease or health problem, and can also alter the perception concerning the benefits versus the barriers to action. Ultimately, it is perception or belief that motivates a person with regard to health habits, compliance behavior, health-seeking behavior, and illness behavior (1).

The health belief model has particular significance when the nurse practitioner is seeking to influence compliance with illness regimens or change health habits, or when the nurse practitioner is working with clients for whom sociocultural factors play a dominant role in influencing illness and wellness beliefs. Some studies have indicated that the greater the perception of barriers to an action, the less likely the person is to take that action. Conversely, fewer perceived barriers to action, in conjunction with the belief that the action is beneficial, correspond with a greater likelihood of action.

Despite the existence of many barriers to action, it is still possible to positively influence health-related behaviors relative to health. The nurse practitioner can promote such change through counseling, health education, and nursing intervention. The following are guidelines for use of the health belief model in clinical practice to influence compliance behavior:

1. Assess the patient's level of knowledge and beliefs concerning a health problem or illness and determine to what extent the client views the problem or illness as a threat.
2. Identify risk factors, sociocultural factors, and other influences that can affect the client's perception of the problem or illness and that can alter the desire to modify or change behavior.
3. Provide health education appropriate to the experience, education, and needs of the client. This may permit more realistic decision making by the client.

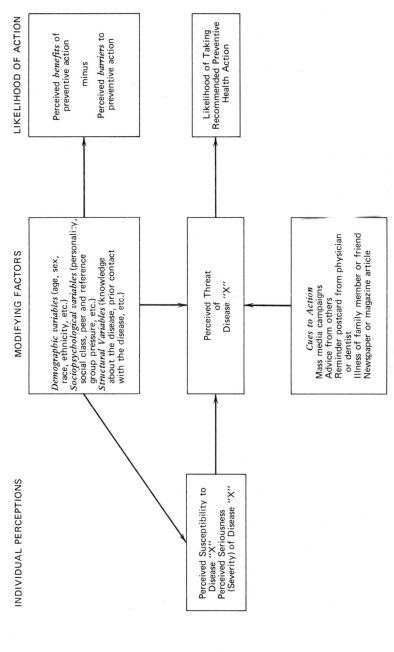

Figure 1.1. The health belief model as predictor of preventive health behavior. (Reprinted with permission from M. H. Becker, [Ed.] *The Health Belief Model and Personal Health Behavior.* Thorofare, N.J.: Charles B. Slack, Inc., 1974.)

4. Discuss with the client the desired behavioral change with particular emphasis on the impact or meaning it will have on the client's lifestyle.
5. Jointly identify the benefits of the desired action or behavior as well as the barriers that will make compliance or change difficult or impossible. Often a written list of benefits versus barriers is helpful for comparison.
6. The client and the nurse practitioner should make a realistic assessment of the feasibility of the desired behavioral change based on the list of barriers versus benefits.
7. After a course of action has been identified, the nurse practitioner can help determine specific and obtainable goals directed toward the desired change.
8. The nurse practitioner can help identify supportive measures that will assist the client in overcoming barriers to the desired action or change; for example, support groups, additional counseling, telephone contacts, or contracting for extra clinic visits. Remember, the greater the barriers to action, the greater the need for structured support, frequent contact, and cues to action.
9. Maintain open communication. To backslide and fail is human. Often health care providers "set up" clients for failure by not hearing their objections or recognizing perceived barriers to action.

QUALITY ASSURANCE

Quality assurance is a process that has as its central goal the promotion of optimal patient care. There is an increasing demand for information concerning the cost-effectiveness of care, whether the care is provided efficiently and effectively, and whether the treatment provided is appropriate to the needs of the client. Great emphasis has been placed on quality assurance by third party financiers of health care in a quest for more accountability. These include both government and private agencies, the Joint Commission on the Accreditation of Hospitals (JCAH), professional associations, and the health care consumer.

Quality assurance has evolved from a method once used to document the efficiency and effectiveness of care to a sophisticated problem solving tool. The concept and process of quality assurance is increasingly applied to the ambulatory care setting. As such it is important that the nurse practitioner be familiar with the organization and components of a quality assurance program.

Quality assurance is now regarded as a method by which health care organizations and professions can upgrade care through the systematic evaluation of client care. The American Nurses Association (ANA) Congress for Nursing Practice model for quality assurance describes the process as a circular one in which evaluations of care are made, the resulting data interpreted as to strengths and weaknesses, and courses of action identified that will improve the future care of clients.

The JCAH standards now require that a hospital quality assurance program emphasize the resolution of problems that will have a significant impact on client care within the facility. A quality assurance program serves not only to provide accountability for the quality of care, but also to provide valuable feedback to the organization and health care staff. This in turn often results in improved client care. The health care professional should be familiar with the components of a quality assurance program in order to become an effective participant.

QUALITY ASSURANCE PROCESS

The first step in implementing a quality assurance program is to identify clearly the area of patient care to be evaluated. While the process can certainly be used to document the efficiency and effectiveness of care already known to be optimal, the process is usually applied to areas in which there is a need to improve the delivery of care. Many facilities set priorities for quality assurance studies according to the areas in which each study could provide feedback. Some areas of study are mandated by federal government financers or the government, as in the case of the Professional Standards Review Organization (PSRO). A quality assurance study can be very broad, including an entire facility or program; or specific, including only one or more aspects of the health care program. The recent trend is to study the quality of care for a specific health care problem, examining all aspects of care. Such a study might include the quality of nursing, medical, respiratory, and laboratory care, as well as other factors contributing to the outcome of the client care for the specific health care problem or condition.

When a quality assurance committee begins an audit, one of the first tasks is identifying the values underlying quality care for the health problem to be studied. Because the definition of quality for a given situation can vary from person to person, it is necessary for the audit committee to define the parameters of quality as it pertains to the audit. Many questions arise at this time, including: what is quality or optimal care for this type of health problem?; what constitutes a valued or desirable outcome?; and what professional and ethical standards will influence decisions concerning quality in this type of case?

The audit committee then develops criteria that describe the various aspects of quality care for this type of problem. Criteria must be measurable and realistic in terms of the setting in which they will be used. Audit criteria for a quality assurance program are developed in order to permit the accurate and valid measurement of quality for the care being evaluated. These criteria can be differentiated to include structural, process, and outcome criteria.

Structural Criteria

Structural criteria focus on the health care facility, organization, staffing, personnel, environment funding, equipment, and/or other prerequisites to optimal client care. The following is an example of a structural criterion:

> The client with viral hepatitis shall be housed in a private room equipped with a sink, toilet, and shower.

Outcome Criteria

Outcome criteria refer to the final results of treatment or care, and are often used to measure the overall success or failure of the care. They focus on the end result of treatment or care rather than the many factors contributing to the care. Outcome criteria are rarely used as the only measure of quality care; the delivery of optimal care to a client does not always guarantee a desirable result, nor does poor client care always result in an undesirable outcome. The following is an example of an outcome criterion:

> Within 10 days after initiating treatment for a urinary tract infection (UTI), the client will be asymptomatic and have sterile urine.

Process Criteria

Process criteria refer to the activities that occur during care and include those that are considered desirable and/or essential to quality care. Process criteria focus on the process of client care as it relates to quality. An example of a process criterion is:

> The client with a UTI shall receive instruction concerning measures that will reduce symptoms and prevent recurrent infections as shown by proper documentation in the health record.

Audit criteria for a quality assurance study normally will include a combination of structure, process, and outcome criteria, all of which reflect the many factors contributing to optimal care.

After the criteria have been identified, the committee determines the standard that will be applied to each criteria. A *standard* is the acceptable degree of variation from the criteria. This is normally expressed as a percentage. Consideration is given to the selection of appropriate methodology and tools necessary for accurate data collection. Data are then collected and measured against the written criteria, and the findings interpreted according to the values associated with quality care.

REGIONAL HEALTH PLANNING

The National Health Planning and Resources Development Act of 1974, Public Law 93-641, resulted in the development of national guidelines for health planning and the creation of state and regional health planning agencies. This legislation recognized the need for a systematic approach to health planning that would be effective at the state and local levels while remaining consistent with national health priorities.

Public Law 93-641, Section 2, notes that "The achievement of equal access to quality health care at a reasonable cost is a priority of the Federal Government." Despite the channeling of large amounts of federal funds into the existing health care system, no corresponding improvement in the accessibility of health services has occurred. Other problems noted in this legislation included the inequitable distribution of health care manpower and resources, the spiraling cost of health care, the lack of a systematic approach to the delivery of health care services, the inappropriate use of the health care system, and a public lack of knowledge regarding personal health practices.

The secretary of the Department of Health and Human Services has designated 203 *health service areas,* or geographic regions, in the United States with each area represented by a nonprofit *health systems agency* (HSA). The secretary is responsible for issuing guidelines for national health policy, which include national health goals and standards for the appropriate supply, distribution, and organization of health services. These guidelines, along with a series of national health priorities outlined in Public Law 93-641, are used by local and state health-planning agencies in the development of a plan consistent with national health policy (2).

In addition to regional HSAs, each state has a *state health planning and development agency* (SHPDA), which is responsible for health planning and resource development as it relates to state government. The SHPDA coordinates with the HSAs within the state and administers a *Certificate of Need* program for new institutional health services. The Certificate of Need program is designed to insure that health care facilities and resources are developed according to the needs of the community, and to prevent unnecessary duplication of services. The agency also conducts public hearings and periodically reviews institutional health services available in the state as to their appropriateness.

In addition to HSA and SHPDA, each state has a *statewide health coordinating council (SHCC)*, which is responsible for coordination among the HSAs in the state, reviewing HSA plans, and controlling applications for federal funds by HSAs and the SHPDA. The SHCC is also responsible for submitting to the governor the state health plan as presented by the SHPDA.

Each HSA is responsible for health care planning within its service area and for the development of adequate health care facilities, resources, and staffing necessary to implement the plan. The governing body of a HSA is composed of consumers and health care providers from the community in a prescribed ratio. The purpose of regional health planning by HSAs is as follows (3):

1. To improve the health status of residents living in the service area.
2. To make quality health care more available and accessible.
3. To increase the continuity of care for residents.
4. To prevent needless duplication of services.
5. To minimize cost increases associated with health care delivery.
6. To maintain competition in the delivery of health services.

The HSA develops a comprehensive health plan consisting of a *health system plan (HSP)* and an *annual implementation plan (AIP)*. These plans are based on careful analysis of the present health of area residents and the available health resources.

The HSP is a long-range plan containing specific goals that will result in improvements in community health as well as available health services. The HSA also develops a short-term AIP. The HSA in collaboration with area, state, and federal organizations seeks changes that will support the long- and short-term plans. The HSA plans generally contain specific objectives designed to improve the overall parameters of health such as communicable disease, infant mortality, and accident rates, as well as goals that will improve the available health services through resource planning.

Other functions of the HSA include reviewing existing health programs in the service area to determine their appropriateness to current needs, making recommendations to the SHPDA concerning certificate of need reviews on projected health care programs, and approving/disapproving proposed use of federal funds at the local level for health care programs.

PROFESSIONAL STANDARDS REVIEW ORGANIZATION

The Professional Standard Review Organization (PSRO) was conceived as a quality assurance program by means of which local physicians might control the quality and cost of federally funded health care through a peer review process.

In the early 1970s Congress focused much concern on the rapidly increasing cost of health care provided under the federal Medicare, Medicaid, and Maternal and Child Health Programs. In 1972 Congress passed Public Law 92–603, which amended the social Security Act to create PSROs. The secretary of the Department of Health, Education and Welfare (now Health and Human Services) designated 203 PSRO areas throughout the United States. Each area is represented by a PSRO composed primarily of local physicians, who are responsible for implementing or overseeing a review process as outlined in the federal PSRO manuals. This responsibility includes determining as to the medical necessity, appropriateness, and quality of care, as well as whether the care is provided economically and in a manner consistent with the client's needs. Ultimately, the PSRO is responsible for the approval or denial of payments for care provided under the auspices of Medicare and Medicaid, thus influencing the quality and cost of care.

PROFESSIONAL STANDARDS REVIEW ORGANIZATION REVIEW PROCESS

PSROs are required to review federally funded health care performed in institutions including hospitals and intermediate- and extended-care facilities. The local PSRO often delegates the actual process of review to the health care facility provided the facility complies with federal PSRO review standards.

The PSRO review process has three components:

1. Concurrent admission certification and continued care review
2. Medical care evaluation studies
3. Analysis of profiles of hospitals, practitioners, and clients

Concurrent review is conducted while the client is undergoing care. This utilization review procedure evaluates the necessity of admission to the facility and the appropriateness of the length of stay. There are two aspects of concurrent PSRO review procedures: (1) Admission certification, and (2) continued care reviews.

Admission Certification

Admission certification consists of a review of the reason for admission in which the admission information is compared against written criteria developed by the PSRO. This results in an evaluation of the appropriateness of the admission to the facility and a determination of a length of stay norm for this admission diagnosis or problem.

Continued Care Review

A *continued care review* is a review performed on or before the client exceeds the initial length of stay established at the time of admission certification. This type of review may result in an extension of the anticipated length of stay when circumstances warrant it, and can trigger a review of the quality of care or result in denial of payment if the admission is unjustifiably lengthy.

Medical Care Evaluation Studies

Medical care evaluation studies are retrospective studies with a purpose and methodology closely resembling a quality assurance audit. Such reviews can be conducted for a specific client in order to examine the quality or appropriateness of care, or can be broadened to include all aspects of health care for a specific client problem or diagnosis.

Profiles of Hospitals, Practitioners, and Clients

Hospital, practitioner, and client profiles involve the compilation of data from concurrent reviews and medical care evaluation studies resulting in the development of profiles for a specific hospital, practitioner, or diagnosis. Such profiles are then used to identify individual institutions or practitioners that are inconsistent with the norm. For example, a profile for a specific diagnosis might display the overall length of stay and usual patient outcome for every hospital in a community. If one hospital had longer stays, and a higher incidence of negative patient outcomes, the facility would be subjected to more intensive review.

PROBLEM-ORIENTED RECORDS

LOGIC OF PROBLEM-ORIENTED RECORDS

Health records have traditionally been organized so that material is filed either consecutively or according to the source of the information, that is, nurse's notes, physician's orders, laboratory, and so on. As source-oriented records become bulky, it is increasingly difficult to locate specific information without reading the entire record. The problem-oriented record (POR) was developed to make it easier to locate in the record information about a specific client problem or diagnosis, to facilitate the communication of information to all members of the health care team, and to display the client data in a logical format.

The POR uses a logical format to document client care and related information. The POR is organized according to specific client problems, thus permitting the rapid location of pertinent information. This system is organized so that all information pertaining to a specific problem or diagnosis is found in one location, including progress notes, laboratory and diagnostic exams, consultant reports, and other pertinent information. For example, the record of a client with hypertension would have a section containing all the information pertaining to this problem.

The POR is composed of the following components: *(1)* initial data base, *(2)* problem list, *(3)* initial plans, *(4)* progress notes, and *(5)* flow sheets.

Initial Data Base

The *initial data base* consists of information gathered pertaining to the client, from which problems can be identified. The data base is normally quite comprehensive and may include a complete health history, physical examination, laboratory and diagnostic examinations, and other related client information. This entire body of information when complete is located in the health record.

Problem List

A *problem list* is a compilation of identified health problems that serves as an index to the health record. The problem list is always located at the front of the record so it is easily visible when the record is opened.

Problems are listed according to the health provider's level of understanding, and may include a diagnosed illness, social and family problems, psychological problems, or abnormal physical findings or symptoms. As problems are listed they receive a number that is used as a reference throughout the health record.

A problem list will normally include space for recording significant major problems as well as minor, self-limiting problems. Problems are categorized according to whether they are active or inactive, along with the date the problem was identified and the date of resolution, where applicable.

Initial Plans

Following the collection of the data base, an *initial plan* is formulated for each problem identified. The initial plan may include treatment recommendations, referrals, client education, and follow-up care.

Progress Notes

In a POR system the *progress notes* are used by practitioners of all disciplines to record progress, list observations, or otherwise document client encounters. Information included when a notation is made on a progress note includes the date, name, and number of problem, and the body of the note, which is usually organized using the *SOAP* format:

S *Subjective data:* what the person tells you—may include symptoms, chief complaint, and review of systems.
O *Objective data:* clinical and diagnostic findings, including physical examination, laboratory and diagnostic data, and behavioral observations.
A *Assessment:* reflects the writer's interpretation of the subjective and objective data to the level of understanding of the problem, for example, diagnosis, symptom(s).
P *Plan:* follow-up treatment, referrals, client education, diagnostic workup, and so on.

Flow Sheet

A *flow sheet* is used to document information that must be collected over a period of time. It can be used to record multiple variables, including vital signs, blood glucose, weight, and laboratory data. A flow sheet easily permits the comparison of serial data and facilitates the recognition of patterns or trends due to its close resemblance to a graph. Flow sheets often are used to record data in the management of diabetes, hypertension, weight control programs, and to monitor changing laboratory values.

STUDY QUESTIONS

Circle all that apply.

1. The health belief model can be useful in clinical practice to explain and predict which of the following?

    a. compliance behavior
    b. potential for high-level wellness
    c. symptoms relating to illness
    d. adaptation to life changes

2. Before a quality assurance audit, criteria are developed that describe various aspects of quality care for the problem being studied. A statement that describes the health care facility, organization, staffing, personnel, funding, equipment, or other prerequisites to optimal patient care is a

    a. process criteria
    b. outcome criterion
    c. structural criterion
    d. management criterion

3. A health systems agency is responsible for the effective health planning and development of health services, manpower, and health facilities within its service area. Which of the following are functions of a health systems agency?

    a. develop health system plan
    b. administer a Certificate of Need program
    c. collect data on health care utilization and community health resources
    d. periodically review institutional health facilities as to appropriateness of services

4. Which of the following review activities are functions of a Professional Standards Review Organization?

    a. admission certification
    b. continued care review
    c. medical care evaluation studies
    d. profiles of hospitals, practitioners, and clients

5. In a problem-oriented record system which of the following is used to record patient data containing multiple variables in a manner that permits serial comparison?

   a. initial data base
   b. problem list
   c. initial plans
   d. progress notes
   e. flow sheet

ANSWERS

1. a
2. c
3. a, b, c, d

4. a, b, c, d
5. e

REFERENCES

1. Becker, M. H. (Ed.) *The health belief model and personal health behavior.* Thorofare, N.J.: Charles B. Slack, 1974.
2. American Hospital Association. *Provisions and legislative intent of Public Law 93–641.* Chicago: American Hospital Association, 1975.
3. National Academy of Science, Institute of Medicine, Committee on Health Planning Goals and Standards. *Health Planning in the United States.* Washington, D.C.: National Academy of Science Press, 1981.

BIBLIOGRAPHY

American Hospital Association, *Provisions and legislative intent of Public Law 93–641.* Chicago: American Hospital Association, 1975.

Becker, M. H. (Ed.). *The health belief model and personal health behavior.* Thorofare, N.J.: Charles B. Slack, 1974.

Creditor, M. C. *Health care planning and development.* Illinois Regional Medical Program, 1974.

Davidson, S. V. S. *PSRO, utilization and audit in patient care.* St. Louis: CV Mosby, 1976.

Egleston, E. M. New JCAH standard on quality assurance. *Nursing Research,* 1980, *29,* 113–14.

Kaplan, K. O., & Hopkins, J. M. *The quality assurance guide—a resource for hospital quality assurance.* Chicago: Joint Committee on the Accreditation of Hospitals, 1980.

Mechanic, D. The stability of health and illness behavior: Results from a 16-year follow-up. *American Journal of Public Health,* 1979, *69,* 1142–45.

National Academy of Science, Institute of Medicine, Committee on Health Planning Goals and Standards. *Health planning in the United States.* Washington, D.C.: National Academy of Science Press, 1981.

Smits, H. L. The PSRO in perspective. *New England Journal of Medicine,* 1981, *305,* 253–59.

CHAPTER 2

THE FAMILY—A SYSTEMS APPROACH TO CARE

Shirley B. Caldwell

As primary care providers, nurse practitioners are in a unique position among health care professionals. They have access to the family as a unit and can know family members as individuals. This available wealth of information is too often bypassed; better care by the provider with increased compliance by the client is often lost when the client, instead of the family, is viewed as the unit of care. Health is affected by environmental and social processes (mainly the family) as well as biological factors (1). Kramer states that "the quality of family life is the most important factor in the health of children" (and adults) (2).

IMPORTANCE OF THE FAMILY SYSTEMS APPROACH

This chapter will show why it is important for the nurse practitioner to view the client as a part of the larger family system, and how illness in one member of the family system can affect the whole family, possibly leading to a crisis. Three possible methods for assessing the family as a system and some basic crisis intervention techniques are also included. As we see the family unit as a whole, we can more easily recognize potential problems and intervene before these problems become acute. As a result, the identified client has a stronger family support system and the family will remain healthier.

Historically, the medical model has focused on the client as the presenting problem. Now, however, some physicians are recognizing that the client has a limited control of events, and that the environment (mainly the family) has a major impact on the health of each of the family members (3–7). To effect change within people, it is often mandatory that changes occur within the larger family unit. Kramer states it this way:

> It is a unique way of thinking about the human condition, a new metaphor, a leap to a different conceptual level. It opens the door to a broader appreciation of the power of families and to a more comprehensive way of understanding changes, i.e. grasping and accepting the family system point of view enables one to look at behavior (and compliance) in a new light. (8)

The family as a system is a modification of general systems theory as first described by von Bertalanffy (9). He defined a *system* as a set of units with relationships among them; these could be one of two types, open or closed. *Open,* or living, systems receive input from the environment surrounding them and are dependent on interaction with the environment for sustenance, growth, and change. In contrast, *closed* systems are sets of units with relationships among them, whose function depends wholly on the system, without input from the environment. Several writers, including Miller and Sedgwick, have applied this theory to families using this definition (10, 11). The family is seen as a complex open system of interdependent parts with each member of the family influencing and being influenced by every other family member. Throughout this process, characteristics of self-regulation are exhibited. In such a family system, self-regulation comes through feedback. Feedback occurs when the output from the system returns in some modified form as input or stimulus to the system. *Feedback* is the means by which the family system informs its members about how to relate to one another and to the external environment, in an attempt to keep the family in a state of homeostasis, or to produce growth. This new concept provides an entirely new way of looking at illness and associated behavior (12).

Today's society is placing significant strains on the family system since the contemporary family is more isolated than in the past, when the members of the extended family shared life together. Childhood and adolescence are also more differentiated and last longer than in earlier years; for example, college students are still financially dependent on their parents even though they are considered adults in other ways. The family is the arena where persons learn values, take on beliefs, absorb attitudes, select role models, and develop as people both positively and negatively. This is the family's legacy to the next generation. Family patterns and beliefs must be understood if the nurse practitioner is to truly plan and know how best to work for the patient's good.

FAMILY SYSTEMS AND CHANGE

The function of the modern family is the socialization and stabilization of adult personalities. In past years, the family performed a variety of other functions; for example, education (now provided by the state) was the responsibility of the family, and family members earned their living together by farming or working in shops (this situation is seldom found today). The marital dyad now lives apart from other adults who might act as support systems during times of crisis. Parents are therefore placed in a structurally unsupported situation, and are more vulnerable to strains on the family system (13). Single-parent families, which are increasing in number each year, are even more susceptible to the stresses found today, since single parents carry the responsibilities of both father and mother. In addition, single parents may be dealing with feelings of grief and emotional suffering accompanying a divorce.

These changes in the family structure—largely in response to wider economic, technological, and cultural changes—are undeniable. They also have had a profound effect on personality formation in children and the later personality stabilization of adults. Sander believes that this has moved the family toward an increasingly private rather than public structure, thus decreasing the wider social control of behavior while increasing its variability (13). He believes this is a possible explanation for the recent increase in the number of referrals to mental health professionals.

The system is further strained by the stress of a long-term or chronic illness of one of the family members. Using the general systems approach, if one part of the system is affected each of the other parts is also affected, with disequilibrium occurring and divorce potential being increased. Miller states:

> The usefulness of systems theory for health professionals who deal with families lies in the concepts which relate to total family functioning. A tendency in the health professions is to treat individual patients for specific physical and psychological problems as if these existed in isolation from families. Frequently, physical and psychological problems are alleviated by medication, surgery, or psychosocial support, but the root cause of the problem within the family system remains untouched.(14)

Too often, health care providers focus only on the physical problem without recognizing its emotional and social impact on all family members. We must remember that increased stress in one member of the system may also lead to infectious illness and symptom formation in other members of the system (15). A person must grow both intrapersonally (inner growth and maturation) and interpersonally, in order to become a healthy individual. A supportive family environment fosters interpersonal growth.

INTERACTIONAL EFFECTS WITHIN FAMILY SYSTEMS

The relationship of parental attitudes and behavior to various forms of stress, illness, and behavior problems in the family has been demonstrated by many researchers (4,5,16–21). However, the impact of disease in causing family stress and dysfunction has been the subject of few systematic studies. Rather, the major focus has been on the family conflict or other family pathology. Arnold et al. has shown that families can be observed, problems identified, and short-term interventions begun (22). These can bring about significant improvements in the family support system, thus greatly benefiting the identified client. Lavigne and Ryan studied the adjustment of the siblings of pediatric hematology, cardiology, and plastic surgery clients with siblings of healthy children (23). They found that siblings of chronically ill children were more likely to show symptoms of irritability and social withdrawal. Further, they gave evidence of much greater fear and inhibition as compared to the siblings of healthy children. After researching the handicapped child and family, Jordan concluded that illness could be described as an entity attacking the family, which is the fundamental social unit (24).

In a study of 25 families with chronically ill children, Taylor found that the single most important problem for the other siblings was the parent–ill child relationship, which resulted in feelings of isolation in the other siblings. However, in families where the healthy children were included in open communication about the problems of the ill child, and had an active part in his or her care, increased emotional growth and empathy in the well siblings developed. Taylor concluded that "through intervention with the entire family, health care providers can maximize such effects and assist the family in coping with their long-term adjustment"(25).

Crain and colleagues also recognized the need to be aware of the effect of an illness of one family member on the behavior of other family members (17). Any illness of a child represents a crisis for the family. One of the predominant sources of stress and conflict in families with a member who has a long-term illness is the time spent in caring for the ill member at the expense of other members. Siblings sense a change in the quality and quantity of time and attention they receive. This frequently leads to feelings of resentment, anger, and/or guilt toward the ill child. Thus it can be understood that families in which the problems of an ill child can be discussed openly, and whose members share in the many tasks that are required and who also feel free to express their own needs, have a decreased chance of other family members being adversely affected. In such families the entire system has the potential for greater growth.

FAMILY SYSTEM DYSFUNCTION

When the family does not meet the psychological needs of individual members, at least one family member will generally provide a signal of *family system dysfunction*. These signals may be in the form of depression, anxiety, anger, and/or somatic complaints such as headaches, gastrointestinal (GI) distress, or muscle spasms (26). Special signals to watch for in children include eneuresis, regression, nightmares, school failure, and aggressive and defiant behavior (27). If the health care provider is focusing only on the identified patient, changes in other members of the family that are not recognized and dealt with will push the family into greater disequilibrium and may ultimately result in a crisis within the family system.

FAMILY SYSTEM CRISIS

Caplan, who has done considerable research in the area, defines family system crisis as occurring:

> when a person faces an obstacle to important life goals, that is, for a time, insurmountable through the utilization of customary methods of problem solving. A period of disorganization ensues, a period of upset, during which many abortive attempts at solution are made.(28)

Crisis can also be defined as a time of both danger and opportunity. The Chinese characters for "crisis" mean both of the above. Crisis becomes a danger when it overwhelms an individual or family to the extent that suicide or a psychotic break may result. However, it may also be a time of opportunity—during times of crisis individuals and families are more open to therapeutic intervention (29).

Crisis can be classified into two categories—*threat,* or a fear of what may happen, and *loss,* for example, loss of a job or of a bodily function, or the death of a relative. The feelings associated with these two categories differ. Crisis precipitated by a threat (perceived or real) results in feelings of acute anxiety, anger, fear, and tension. Crisis resulting from a loss is usually manifested by depression, masked anger, withdrawal, hostility, and/or guilt. People in crisis usually exhibit a decreased perception of incoming information. Their ability to solve problems is impaired, and they are less aware of alternative options. These people also have a feeling of being immobilized and are unable to master new tasks. They also have a decreased sense of personal effectiveness and creativity. As a result, the capacity to make constructive decisions, is very limited, and these people turn inward, becoming self-occupied (30). The primary care provider needs to be constantly aware of the signs and symptoms indicating that all is not well in the family system. Families that have a member with a chronic or terminal illness should be monitored closely, and support and/or crisis intervention initiated if indicated.

Management

The primary care provider can offer the help that many clients need in a crisis situation. Loss is a part of every life; therefore, clients should be allowed to grieve. If you as the primary care provider are also feeling grief, give yourself permission to express it in an appropriate manner.

Some somatic signs of grief that the client may exhibit include deep sighing and increased physical complaints; feelings of unreality may also occur. The client and family should be reassured that this is not abnormal. They can also be encouraged to talk about memories, and even to idealize the terminally ill or deceased person.

Great self-awareness is needed on the part of the helper in a crisis situation. "I perceive . . ." statements are helpful for giving feedback. Confrontation should be used with restraint. The primary care provider should help family members to restructure their environment first, and then to deal with their feelings. Only after these two areas are dealt with should the underlying problems be discussed. Following up on "feeling" clue words while remaining alert to the anxiety level that is shown is another way the primary care provider can assist clients in a crisis situation.

Client anxiety may be eased by encouraging deep breathing, perhaps modeling such breathing for the client; speaking in a lower tone of voice; relaxing yourself and encouraging the client to do the same; and, if appropriate, using touch to make contact. The client may be helped to explore new options and given encouragement, reassurance, and hope whenever possible. A genuinely caring provider has much to offer clients in crisis.

According to Aguilera and Messick, crisis intervention offers potential for growth because families are believed to be more open to change during a crisis than at any other time, and to learning new ways of coping (29). Another reassuring aspect of crisis is that it is time limited. Most crises have been passed or resolved within two months, so that the primary health provider must not postpone action when a family is in crisis, but rather provide the support and help in problem solving needed immediately. The focus needs to be on the "here and now" for crisis situations. Families in which major interpersonal problems exist may benefit from referral. The goal of the nurse practitioner should be to prevent emotional handicaps in all members of the family.

ASSESSMENT OF FAMILY SYSTEMS

How then can a nurse practitioner in a primary care setting assess the family system? There are several ways in which this can be done; three different approaches will be reviewed at this time.

FAMILY APGAR

The first and most concise measure to be reviewed is Smilkstein's *Family APGAR*. This is a brief screening questionnaire designed to test five areas of family functioning and provide a "data base that will reflect a patient's point of view of the functional state of his or her family"(31). The five areas fit the acronym APGAR—*adaptability, partnership, growth, affection,* and *resolve*. Briefly defined, these are:

Adaptation. How are intra- and extrafamilial resources used in problem solving during times of family crisis?

Partnership. Are decision making and nurturing responsibilities shared by family members? (Includes family members' satisfaction with communication and problem solving.)

Growth. Are family members achieving physical and emotional maturation and self-fulfillment through mutual support and guidance? (Includes members' satisfaction with the freedom available to change roles.)

Affection. Are there caring and loving relationships among family members?

Resolve. Is there a commitment to devote time and/or energy to other family members as needed for their physical and emotional nurturing?

These five areas are included in a questionnaire that features five questions to be answered by one of three options: "almost always" (three points), "some of the time" (two points), or "hardly ever" (one point). This questionnaire is applicable to either nuclear or alternative life-style families i.e. communal, homosexual or heterosexual committed relationships. A validity index is being established.

Smilkstein recommends the use of this questionnaire whenever a patient appears to be in crisis. She believes that information obtained from the patient about how family members eat, sleep, and carry out home, school, and job responsibilities can alert the health care provider to the need to evaluate the family function in greater detail. In such cases, the five areas can be covered by the use of open-ended questions such as:

Adaptation.   How has your family helped you in the past, or you them? Is there anyone in your community that has helped you in the past?

Partnership.   How do members of your family talk with each other about such things as vacations, finances, large purchases, or financial problems?

Growth.   How have family members changed across the years? Has it been easy to leave home? Do you feel that you have your family's support in your changes?

Affection.   How do members of your family show their affection, love, anger, or sorrow?

Resolve.   How do members of your family share their time, money, and space?

Such questions can lead to more detailed information than the questionnaire method but do require more time to complete: thus the health care provider needs to decide which method(s) is (are) best in each situation.

Three types of patient situations that seem appropriate for the use of the Family APGAR are suggested: one situation involves gathering functional information about the family when planning home care for a client. Base-line data about family functioning can aid the provider in planning for care in the home. If the family has a high score, the provider could assume that the family would more likely adapt to the client's illness and needs; however, if the score was low, the provider may need to take a closer look at family interaction before sending the client home.

Second, the Family APGAR is used to gather base-line data during the first appointment with a client. Such an encounter allows the health care provider to gain insight into the family and permits the family members to meet the health care provider. It is recommended that thereafter the test be given periodically, for example, every five years, to maintain an understanding of the family as a system.

A third situation for which the Family APGAR is applicable is when a family is in trouble or when a client reports a crisis. This should be taken as an indication that the family's past coping skills may not be adequate for the current problem. In such a case, the author suggests that if a client scores 0 to 1 in some area, then the health care provider could follow up with an appropriate open-ended question in that specific area. Case studies demonstrating how the Family APGAR has been used in each of these three areas are provided in Smilkstein's study.

Family Functioning Index

The second method of assessing family functioning is that developed by Pless and Satterwhite. They recognized that the need to understand the family unit "is of pervasive importance in many aspects of child health. Nevertheless, the knowledge a doctor has of a family is often fragmentary" (32). Pless and Satterwhite felt that this was a liability in the planning of realistic care for the client, so they developed an instrument that could be administered in a clinic setting—the *Family Functioning Index* (FFI). Categories covered by the FFI include the following and are rated using a Likert scale (33).

Marital Satisfaction.   Feelings about your marriage, standard of living, love, affection, companionship.

Frequency of Disagreements.   From the spouse's perspective, did the household have more, the same, or fewer disagreements than other families that he or she knows?

Happiness.   Overall, is your family happier than most others you know, about the same, or less happy?

Communication.   Is your spouse an easy person to talk to when things are bothering you?

Weekends Together.   What sort of things does your family do on weekends?

Problem Solving.   Remembering the most important problem you had as a family this past year, did you discuss this with your spouse?*(33)

*A copy of the complete questionnaire is available from Pless and Satterwhite. I.B. Pless-formerly University of Rochester, Rochester, N.Y., now Montreal Children's Hospital, Montreal, Quebec, Canada.

The range for a total possible score is from 0 to 35. The higher the scores, the higher the level of family functioning. The validity of this questionnaire was tested in three different types of settings using independent ratings by various professionals, correlated with the parent's ratings. The conclusions were that the FFI has a "reasonable degree of validity and reliability"(34).

Applications for use of such an index should be considered in cases where greater knowledge about a family system is needed in planning care for any aged client. The authors believe that this measure, or a similar one, is likely to be of greater value than the assessment of social class, family size, ethnicity, or religion. It can also be used as a means of predicting the psychological well-being of chronically ill and healthy children (35). If the nurse practitioner, using the previous six areas of assessing the level of family functioning, finds a low rating for a family in which there is also a child with a chronic disease, increasing behavioral problems in the ill child might also be found. The nurse practitioner would then explore intervention strategies to decrease mental health and physical disturbances in the ill child and in other family members.

Assessment of Family Function

The third family evaluation method discussed has just recently been developed by Florence Roberts (36). This model uses both the provider and client when assessing the needs of the client. Roberts sees the client as being more aware of certain needs and knowing more about previous responses than any health care provider. She believes clients need to be given as much control as possible; to be encouraged to assume responsibility, not abdicate their bodies to the health provider's control. Both client and health care provider have expertise, but in different areas. Only when the client becomes critically ill does the health care provider take over the care of the client. Therefore, the health care provider and the client (family) together evaluate the family's functions and mutually select which of the client's needs each will be responsible for. Benoliel also believes that by using total family interviewing the tremendous and variable influences of family relationships can be determined more easily (37).

In using Roberts' model, the family is jointly assessed according to the following functional categories:

1. Management (power, finances, rules, relationships with community, schools, police, and so on, future plans)
2. Boundaries (individual, generational, protective role, and family)
3. Communication (are messages congruent, not manipulative; do they show positive and negative feelings?)

4. Emotional—supportive (mutual positive regard, willingness to deal with conflict, family members have freedom to grow as individuals)
5. Socialization (healthy, developing children; mutual interaction; parents experiencing parental satisfaction)

Each item is then rated at a certain level:

Level I.   Current needs are met; no help is needed; problems are identified; health care provider acts as a resource.

Level II.   Current needs are met but potential problems are identified; health care provider is an educator and facilitator.

Level III.   Current needs are not being met; obvious problems are identified. The health care provider works collaboratively with the client to resolve the problem.

Level IV.   There is social, psychological, or physical danger—a crisis situation. The health care provider acts in a protective role.

From this joint (health care provider and family) assessment, needs are identified. If needs as perceived by the provider are not seen as needs by the client and do not result in a life-threatening crisis, Roberts feels that expending the provider's energy in trying to meet such needs is probably a waste of time. She believes that the client should assume the major responsibility for assessing his or her needs except where the client lacks the necessary knowledge, experience, or ability to do so. The more the family is involved, the greater the motivation will be to work toward change.

As previously identified, the role of the health care provider is determined by the level of needs. If the family can manage with some basic educational instruction, then the provider should educate, not attempt to make the family dependent on the provider. The family should be encouraged to assume as much control as possible. A more complete description including a model can be found in Roberts' original article. This model has been written particularly for nurse practitioners but is applicable to all health care providers.

Thus, it can be seen that families that have identified potential or real problems in their family systems may only need to have family communication channels opened. The health care provider, by bringing real problems into the problem solving process, functions as a facilitator or consultant while the family does the basic problem solving. Some educational guidance may be helpful, but the family is motivated to make changes to strengthen its own system. Some families may need homework assignments, follow-up sessions to monitor progress, and support and reassurance. Insight and new ideas may also come through parent support groups, family counseling sessions, or assigned readings pertinent to the problem areas. Each family is unique. Therefore, the nurse practitioner is urged to be sensitive to the family system, to take time to assess the system, to plan and attempt intervention, and to evaluate results. Remember, the greatest asset any health care provider brings to a poorly functioning family system is a genuine sense of caring.

By using these additional assessments, the primary health care provider can be alert to other potential problems that may develop or intervene before a particular problem becomes acute.

The health care provider is urged to consult the works listed in the reference section.

STUDY QUESTIONS

The K. family, which consists of Mr. and Mrs. K. and their two children, Sharon, 10 years and David, 8 years, are known to the Primary Care Clinic because of David and his diabetes, diagnosed one year ago. David comes in regularly, since his diabetes is fairly labile, especially when his meals are not eaten regularly or his amount of exercise changes significantly. The nurse practitioner has been trying to educate both David and his mother about diabetes. The management of David has been discussed, including ways of adapting the restrictions of the diabetic into their family life-style. The father and Sharon are rarely seen and have been assumed to be doing well. However, at the last visit, when David and his mother were in, the nurse practitioner incidentally asked about "the rest of the family" and Mrs. K. replied, "I guess they're O.K. I'm so involved with David and his diabetes I guess I haven't paid much attention." When the nurse practitioner heard this, she realized that there were probably other problems in the family, so she suggested that the whole family come for the next visit.

The following week, the nurse practitioner was pleased to find the entire K. family in the waiting room. After David's diabetes was assessed, the family was asked to come into the conference room. The session began by reviewing diabetes and its management, and asking the family if they had questions. Then the family was asked how they felt David's diabetes had affected them. The responses were as follows:

Mrs. K.: "I am really on edge. There always seems to be something I need to keep reminding David about. I am afraid to go out with my friends as before because the school might call saying David has a reaction and they need me; or I'm fixing special food. Our family is just not being much of a family anymore."

David: "I hate all those shots. I don't see why I have diabetes and Mom's always on to me about something."

Sharon: "Well, at least they notice you! No one ever seems to have any time for me any more. Mother is so busy with David and Daddy is away so much."

Mr. K.: "Why, Sharon, I didn't know you felt like that. I guess one of the main ways David's diabetes has hit me is in my pocketbook. All these extra visits, blood tests, and medicine really take a lot of extra money, so I'm working another job. Seems like I'm not home much and when I am, my wife here is complaining about something. Sharon has also been having trouble in school and is getting into all sorts of trouble at home. She used to be such a sweet little kid."

Circle all that apply.

1. In assessing the K. family, the member who is probably closest to a crisis is:

   a. mother
   b. father
   c. Sharon
   d. David

2. An appropriate response for the nurse practitioner to make after listening to the family would be:

   a. "You shouldn't let this bother you so much, since David seems to be doing well now."
   b. "David's diabetes has certainly messed up your family."
   c. "It seems to me that each one of you is having a different kind of problem that you feel began with David's diabetes."
   d. "It sounds to me like each of you is angry or frustrated. Tell me some more about these feelings, then let's look at some possible solutions."

3. Some indications of potential crisis in the K. family include:

   a. increased tension
   b. anger
   c. increased verbalization
   d. decreased awareness of others needs
   e. increased somatic complaints

4. Using Smilkstein's Family APGAR scale, which areas would probably receive the lowest ratings when assessing the K. family?

   a. adaptation
   b. partnership
   c. growth
   d. affection
   e. resolve

5. Family intervention for the K. family needs to include:

   a. opening communication among all members
   b. helping parents plan time to be with Sharon
   c. recognizing and accepting current feelings felt by each family member
   d. group problem solving
   e. scheduling a follow-up family session in about three months

ANSWERS

1. c
2. d
3. a, b, d

4. a, b, c, d, e
5. a, b, c, d, e

REFERENCES

1. Haggerty, R. J., Roghmann, K. J. & Pless, I. B. *Child health and the community*. New York: John Wiley & Sons, 1975.
2. Kramer, C. H. *Becoming a family therapist*. New York: Human Sciences Press, 1980.
3. Sander, F. M. *Individual and family therapy: Toward an integration*. New York: Jason Aronson, 1979.
4. Minuchen, S., Baker, L., Rosman, B. L. A conceptual model of psychosomatic illness in children: Family organization and family therapy. *Archives of General Psychiatry*, 1975, *32*, 1031–1038.
5. Pless, I. B., & Satterwhite, B. A measure of family functioning and its application. *Social Science Medicine*, 1973, *7*, 613.
6. Baker, L., Levine, A. G., & Patterson, G. R. Changes in sibling behavior following family intervention. *Journal of Consulting Clinical Psychology*, 1975, *43*(5), 683–688.

7. Smilkstein, G. The Family APGAR: A proposal for a family function test and its use by physicians. *Journal of Family Practice,* 1978, *6*(6), 1231–1239.

8. Kramer, *op. cit.,* pp. 50–51.

9. Von Bertalanffy, L. *General systems theory.* New York: George Braziller, 1968.

10. Miller, J. C. Systems theory and family psychotherapy. *Nursing Clinics of North America,* 1971, *6*(3), 395–406.

11. Sedgwick, R. *Family mental health.* St. Louis: C V Mosby, 1981.

12. Haley, J. *Leaving home.* New York: McGraw-Hill, 1980.

13. Sander, F. M. *Individual and family therapy: Toward an integration.* New York: Jason Aronson, 1979.

14. Miller, J. R., & Janosik, E. H. *Family-focused care.* New York: McGraw-Hill, 1980.

15. Pratt, L. *Family structure and effective health behavior: The energized family.* Boston: Houghton Mifflin, 1976.

16. Koski, M. L., Ahlas, A., & Kumento, A. A psychosomatic follow-up study of childhood diabetics. *Acta Paedopsychiatry,* 1976, *42,* 12–26.

17. Crain, A. J., Sussman, M. B., & Weil, B. W. Family interaction, diabetes, and sibling relationships. *International Journal of Social Psychiatry,* 1966, *12,* 35–43.

18. Etzwiler, D. D., & Sines, L. K. Juvenile diabetes and its management: Family, social and academic implications. *Journal of American Medical Association,* 1962, *181*(4), 304–308.

19. Swift, C. F., Seidman, F., & Stein, H. Adjustment problems in juvenile diabetes. *Psychosomatic Medicine,* 1967, *29,* 555–576.

20. Stierlin, H., Rucker-Embden, I., Wetzel, N. *The first interview with the family.* New York: Brunner/Mazel, 1980.

21. Quint, J. C. The developing diabetic identity: A study of family influence. In M. V. Batey (Ed.), *Communicating nursing research: Methodological issues in research.* Boulder, Colo.: *Western Interstate Commission on Higher Education,* 1970, *3,* 14–32.

22. Arnold, J. E., Levine, A. G., & Patterson, G. R. Changes in sibling behavior following family intervention. *Journal of Consulting Clinical Psychology,* 1975, *43*(5), 683–688.

23. Lavigne, J. V., & Ryan, M. Psychologic adjustment of siblings of children with chronic illness. *Pediatrics,* 1979, *63,* 616–627.

24. Jordan, T. E. Research on the handicapped child and the family. *Merrill–Palmer Quarterly,* 1962, *8,* 240–252.

25. Taylor, S. C. The effects of chronic childhood illnesses upon well siblings. *Maternal-Child Nursing Journal,* 1980, *9*(2), 109–116.

26. Lantz, J. E. *Family and marital therapy: A transactional approach.* New York: Appleton-Century-Crofts, 1978.

27. Smith, M. H. Challenges of psychological care. In D. Fatchman & G. Foley (Eds.), *Nursing care of the child with cancer.* New York: Little, Brown (in press).

28. Caplan, G. *An approach to community mental health.* New York: Grune & Stratton, 1961.

29. Aguilera, D. C., & Messick, J. M. *Crisis intervention* (4th ed.): St. Louis: CV Mosby, 1982.

30. Calhoun, G. On the spot counseling techniques in crisis. *Workshop presentation at Tennessee State University,* Nashville, TN, 1980.

31. Smilkstein, G., *op. cit.,* p. 1231.

32. Pless, I. B., & Satterwhite, B. A measure of family functioning and its application. *Social Science Medicine,* 1973, *7,* 613.

33. *Ibid.,* p. 614.

34. *Ibid.,* p. 618.

35. Pless, I. B., & Satterwhite, B. Family functioning and family problems. In R. J. Haggarty, K. J. Roghmann, & I. B. Pless (Eds.), *Child health and the community.* New York: John Wiley & Sons, 1975.

36. Roberts, F. B. Assessment of family function. In I. Clements & F. B. Roberts (Eds.), *Family Health: Theoretical Approaches to Nursing Care.* New York: John Wiley & Sons, 1983.

37. Benoliel, J. Q. The developing diabetic identity: a study of family influence. *Communicating Nursing Research,* 1970, *3,* 14–27.

CHAPTER **3**

WELL CHILD CARE

Rosalie Hammond Pazulinec

Well child care, also referred to as child health supervision, is considered an extremely valuable component of pediatric health care. The objectives of well child care are:

1. Prevention of disease
2. Early detection and treatment of disease
3. Guidance for the parents in the psychosocial aspects of child rearing (1)

Well child care (as opposed to illness care) has the advantage of being truly preventive and family oriented. It provides for contact with families at strategic points in family development as well as providing for continuity and the development of trust through repeated visits to a health care provider. Because childhood nutritional and infectious diseases have become less important health problems for the majority of children in this country, more effort can be focused on parental support and on guidance of child care during health care visits. This support can be especially valuable to today's young families who no longer have the extended family available to them.

There is evidence in both the pediatric and nursing literature that supports the provision of well child care by nurse practitioners. Not only have nurse practitioners been found to provide as high a quality of well child care as pediatricians, but parental acceptance of nurse practitioners has been positive as well (2–5). The following sections provide a synopsis of information that should be useful to nurse practitioners involved in the care of well children and their families.

GUIDELINES

The American Academy of Pediatrics (AAP) has established standards for well child care (see Table 3.1) and suggests that these be used as a guideline rather than as rigid criteria for care (6). The standards were originally established by AAP in 1967 and were based on expert opinion rather than empirical data. Because the number of visits necessary to provide adequate well child care had not been established, a study was undertaken to look into this issue. The study revealed that less than the recommended visits is probably adequate provided that immunizations can be given at recommended times (4). The AAP recommendations are now more flexible and place increased emphasis on meeting the individual needs of each child. The AAP has also described the following situations that may indicate the need for additional visits.

1. First born or adopted children or those not with natural parents
2. Parents with a particular need for education and guidance
3. Disadvantaged social or economic environment
4. The presence or possibility of perinatal disorders, such as low birth weight, congenital defects, or familial disease
5. Acquired illness or previously identified disease or problems (6)

In general, health care providers should adhere to a schedule of visits that provides for adequate screening, prevention, and early detection of illness, as well as time for parental guidance and support. Whether or not one follows the AAP guidelines is left to the individual practitioner.

IMMUNIZATIONS

The administration of immunizations to infants and children is one of the truly preventive aspects of well child care. Immunizations do not necessarily have to be administered during a regularly scheduled visit, but can be given

Table 3.1. Recommendations for Preventive Health Care

Age	2–4 Wks.	2–3 Mos.	4–5 Mos.	6–7 Mos.	9–10 Mos.	12–15 Mos.	16–19 Mos.	23–25 Mos.	36–37 Mos.	5–6 Yrs.	8–9 Yrs.	11–12 Yrs.	13–15 Yrs.	16–21 Yrs.
History														
Initial							At first visit							
Interval							At each visit							
Measurements														
Height and weight							At each visit							
Head circumference	✓	✓		✓		✓		✓						
Blood pressure									✓	✓	✓	✓	✓	✓
Sensory screening														
Sight	✓✓	✓		✓✓					✓✓ OR	✓✓ OR	✓	✓	✓	✓
Hearing	✓	✓		✓✓					✓✓ OR	✓✓ OR	✓		✓	
Developmental appraisal									At each visit					

Physical exam · · · · · · · · · · · · · · At each visit · · · ·

Procedures

Immunization ✓ · ✓ ✓ · · · ✓ · · · · ✓ · · ✓ · · · · · ·

Tuberculin test · · · · · ✓ · · · · · · ✓ · · · · · ·

Hematocrit or
Hgb · · ✓ · · ✓ · OR ✓ · · ✓ · · ·

Urinalysis · · · · · ✓ · · · ✓ · · ✓ · · ·

Urine culture (girls only) · · · · · · ✓ · · · · ✓ · · ·

Discussion and
counseling · · · · · · · · At each visit · · ·

Dental screening · · · · · · · · · · At each visit · · ·

Initial dentist's
exam · · · · · · · · · · · ✓ · ·

Source: Reproduced with permission from *Standards of Child Health Care*, 3rd edition, 1977. Copyright American Academy of Pediatrics 1977.

Table 3.2. Routine Immunizations

Age at Administration[a]	Types of Immunizations		
	DPT	Oral Polio	Measles, Mumps, Rubella
2 months (6–8 wks)	X	X	
4 months	X	X	
6 months	X	X	
15 months[b]			X
18 months	X	X	
4–6 years	X	X	
14–16 years and every 10 years thereafter	Td[c]		

Note: Smallpox vaccine is no longer given, even for foreign travel.

[a]Should an infant miss one of the primary series of DPT (diphtheria–pertussis–tetanus) or polio vaccines, there is no need to start over, but to continue with the primary series (first three doses) as scheduled. Should an adult be unimmunized, the primary series would follow a slightly different schedule.

[b]A TB (tuberculin) skin test is usually given at this time. It is no longer required to give them yearly due to a decreased incidence of the disease.

[c]After the child is 6 years old, DPT is no longer administered to the increasing severity of reaction to the pertussis vaccine with age. After age 6, Td (tetanus-diphtheria) is used instead.

by a nurse through an office or health department according to routine schedules. Parents should be informed of the nature and value of the routine immunizations, and infants should be started at the earliest possible age according to the schedule (see Table 3.2). Although today one does not hear of outbreaks of polio, whooping cough, or diptheria, the organisms that cause these diseases are still present in the environment. They could cause significant illness or death to infants and young children if large numbers of people fail to become immunized.

In general, most vaccines can safely be given simultaneously at separate sites. A contraindication to inactivated vaccines, such as diphtheria, pertussis, and tetanus vaccines (DPT) would be a previous severe reaction to the vaccine. Contraindications to live attenuated vaccines generally include leukemia, lymphoma, or generalized malignancy; an immunosuppressed state, such as occurs with corticosteroids, antimetabolites, and radiation therapy; a severe febrile illness (a cold is not a contraindication); or recent (up to three months) injection of human immune globulin (7). Pregnancy is a contraindication to live attenuated vaccines because of the theoretical risk of exposure to the fetus. However, children of pregnant mothers can and should receive measles and rubella vaccines.

DPT is given as a combined inactivated form and administered intramuscularly. Adverse reactions to this range from mild to severe and generally consist of slight fever and local erythema at the injection site for a few hours.

Almost 30% of infants have a more pronounced local reaction and fever for a longer period. Uncommonly severe reactions can occur, consisting of (1) seizures within 72 hours after injection; (2) shock-like syndrome (rare with U.S. vaccine); (3) persistent unconsolable screaming (continuous for five hours and intermittent for 12 hours); and (4) irreversible brain damage or death (8). If any of the severe reactions occur, no further pertussis vaccine should be given, and only tetanus-diphtheria (Td), if the child is over 6 years old, administered for subsequent doses in the series. Occasionally, it has been reported that a sterile chronic granuloma has occurred at the injection site. Children older than 6 years who have never been immunized should receive DT for 2 doses at six to eight week intervals, followed by a reinforcing dose in one year. At the time of administration of DPT and oral polio, parents should be informed of the common side effects and told to return if more severe reactions occur. It is often suggested that parents give the infant an appropriate oral dose of acetaminophen or aspirin after immunization to relieve discomfort. Oral polio is a live attenuated trivalent vaccine that has few side effects in its present form. However, paralysis has occured (*rarely*) and would be more likely to occur in immune-deficient persons (9).

Measles, mumps, and rubella are all live viral vaccines that should be given to children at 15 months of age or older for an adequate host-immune response to occur. Mumps is considered lower priority than the other aforementioned vaccines but is stressed especially for preadolescent or young adult males. The measles vaccine (usually given in combination with rubella and mumps) has greatly reduced the incidence of this disease and, therefore, the high rate of complications that resulted from it, such as otitis media, pneumonia, and encephalitis. The reaction to measles vaccine is usually a mild fever that occurs about six days after immunization and lasts up to five days. Transient rashes are rare, and more severe reactions (encephalopathy) have occurred in only 1 per 1 million doses (10). Rubella vaccine was developed to aid in the prevention of rubella infection in early pregnancy. It is an effective vaccine and should be given at 12 months of age (15 months with combination vaccine) or older. Side effects have occurred from 2 to 10 weeks after immunization and have included rash, lymphadenopathy, and arthralgias. The joint manifestations are more frequent and severe in women than in children (11).

Special attention should be paid to the immunization status of children with chronic disease, or mental and/or physical handicaps. Because the practitioner's main focus is often on the children's problems, their primary care occasionally has been neglected and they have not been adequately immunized in spite of numerous visits to physicians or health care facilities. In addition to the routine immunizations, special vaccines, such as Pneumovax and influenza should be considered for these children, depending on their problems.

SCREENING

Screening in a pediatric practice is aimed at the early detection and treatment of disease. It becomes an integral aspect of the well child visit and includes activities and procedures, such as a screening history and physical, specific laboratory tests, developmental appraisal, and vision testing. To adequately screen infants and children, one needs to have knowledge of normal growth and development as well as common disorders of infancy and childhood. A general knowledge of hereditary disorders, environmental hazards, and populations at risk for various problems is necessary. In general, screening should be done only for disorders that can be accurately diagnosed and for which early detection and treatment is likely to be beneficial. The time span from onset of a disorder (asymptomatic) to the development of symptoms or disability helps one to decide the frequency of screening.

Health care providers should be familiar with community resources and have knowledge of definitive diagnostic and appropriate remediation services available to a patient being screened for a particular disorder. It should be the responsibility of well child care providers to see that appropriate screening is available either in their setting or elsewhere in the community and that adequate follow-up services are also available. Table 3.1 includes screening activities that are recommended as guidelines by the American Academy of Pediatrics.

GENERAL SCREENING ACTIVITIES

General screening is included in routine health care throughout the life-span of normal children and adults. The neonate should be screened for phenylketonuria (PKU) and hypothyroidism. During infancy, one of the parameters evaluated at each visit, through the measurement of head circumference, height, and weight, is physical growth and development. Head circumference should be measured at routine visits until the child is at least two years of age, when head growth should be near completion. Measurements of height and weight at separate intervals give an indication of the rate of growth, so that aberrations can be picked up early. These measurements should be recorded on a standard growth chart for accurate interpretation. Problems with growth can be related to numerous factors, for example, nutritional, emotional, metabloic, and congenital defect and the etiology should be determined after detection of growth problems.

The screening history and physical examination should be conducted at each well child visit. Various components of the history and physical should be performed at different visits, depending on the child's age and his or her degree of risk for particular disorders as determined by the history, ethnic origin, or socioeconomic status. During the initial and interval histories, the practitioner should gain knowledge of the perinatal period, family history, developmental status through appraisal of milestones, parental concerns, the home environment, and past illnesses. This information will help pinpoint high risk areas, and help the practitioner focus the discussion during the visit so that possible problem areas will not be overlooked. For example, a child with a history of a traumatic perinatal course would deserve more attention to developmental screening, and the parents should be told that this area will be watched and that their concerns will not be taken lightly.

Numerous problems can easily be detected during the physical exam. Orthopedic problems, such as congenital hip dislocation and scoliosis, are screened by exam. Newborns should be screened for hip disease by both the Ortolani and Barlow maneuvers, with a follow-up exam by hip abduction at subsequent visits until the child begins to walk. Neonates should be screened also for retinoblastoma by examining the eyes for the anatomical red reflex. Other problems that can be uncovered in the neonatal period by the physical examination include cardiac disease through auscultation for murmurs and palpation of pulses (especially femoral), inguinal hernias, and certain genetic syndromes. The screening exam should, of course, be individualized according to risk.

SPECIFIC SCREENING PROCEDURES

Cardiac Disease.   Screening for cardiac disease should be done throughout childhood—twice in the first six months when congenital heart disease might become evident, at school entry, and during preadolescent and adolescent visits to rule out acquired disease. Blood pressure should be taken at 3 years, 5 years, and 10 years, and again in adolescence (12).

Anemia.   Anemia is a disorder that can be accurately screened for through determination of the hematocrit or hemoglobin. Most congenital anemias (sickle cell, thalassemia) can be detected by 6 months of age, and iron deficiency anemia is most likely to occur between 8 and 12 months of age. Therefore, most infants should have a hematocrit at about 9 months. An infant in this age group would be considered anemic with a hemaglobin of less than 10 grams or a hematocrit of less than 30%. It should be remembered that anemia is a symptom of disease in many cases, and the etiology of the anemia (i.e., hereditary, nutritional, chronic illness) needs to be determined before any therapy can be instituted.

Lead Intoxication. Although lead intoxication is not as prevalent as was previously thought, there are certain at risk populations that would require screening. Children with known environmental exposure or those living in areas where houses were built before World War II should be screened sometime in the period between 18 months and 5 years when they are at highest risk. Screening is done by blood lead determination or nonspecifically with free erythrocyte porphyrins (1).

Tuberculosis. Screening for tuberculosis is not done as frequently as in the past due to a decreased prevalence of the disease in many areas. However, inner city children and children at high risk due to geographical location should be screened at ages 1 year, 3 years, and at school entry. Screening can be done with the Tine (old tuberculin) or the Mono-Vacc test, but should be followed by the intradermal Mantoux—intermediate purified protein derivative (IPPD)—when results are positive. Any child suspected of exposure or illness should be screened with an IPPD (1, 12).

Genitourinary. The need to screen for genitourinary problems has not been firmly established. At the present time, it is strongly recommended that all children be screened for proteinuria (dipstik method) usually once in the preschool, preadolescent, and adolescent age groups, and that girls be screened for bacteriuria in the preschool period by some type of culture method. Screening for pyuria and glycosuria has not been found to be worthwhile (6, 12).

SCREENING OF SPECIAL SENSES

Because adequate hearing and vision are important aspects in normal growth and development, screening of vision and hearing is an essential component of well child care and is often carried out through community agencies (public health, school). Newborns should be tested grossly for sight by checking the blink and pupillary reflexes to light. Older infants should be watched for their ability to fix on and follow objects. They should be screened for strabismus by the cover test method and by observing for a symmetrical corneal light reflex. Infants suspected of strabismus or a visual acuity problem should be evaluated by an ophthalmologist. Visual acuity in older infants and children should be screened during the preschool period and again between the ages of about 10 to 13 years. This can be done with Snellen-type charts. Referral should be made for vision of 20/50 or greater.

Normal hearing is essential for language development, and therefore, any suspicion of poor hearing should be evaluated, preferably by an audiologist. All children should be screened by pure-tone audiometry before school entry. This is often offered in the community, but can be done as an office procedure. Younger infants and children who have a history of recurrent otitis or meningitis, who have abnormal language development, who have a positive family history of deafness, or whose parents have a concern about hearing, should be evaluated. Screening tests for younger children have been developed and can be carreid out in a practice setting. These include the Hardy test for 8 to 12 month-olds, which presents standardized sounds to a child to test for the ability to localize sound. Three and 4 year-olds can be given the Verbal Auditory Screening for Children (VASC) (12).

Normal language development should begin with babbling at 4 months; echolalic language (e.g., bye-bye-bye) at 9 or 10 months; single words at 1 year; and speech in phrases at 18 months to 2 years. By 3 years of age, 90% of a child's speech should be understandable. If a child does not follow this pattern, both a developmental and audiologic evaluation is recommended. Practitioners should be warned that both vision and hearing disorders could be manifested as developmental delay and they should be aware of this before the child becomes inaccurately labeled as "delayed" or "retarded."

DEVELOPMENTAL SCREENING

Developmental screening cannot be performed alone according to a pre-scribed schedule but becomes an integral aspect of each well child visit, based on a thorough knowledge of normal growth and development. It is beyond the scope of this chapter to discuss the developmental information needed for adequate screening and assessment, but certain aspects of screening for developmental problems can be described. It should be re-membered that developmental changes (physical, emotional, cognitive) that occur are both quantitative and qualitative. Development occurs in predicta-ble, sequential patterns with a wide variation of observable behaviors con-sidered to be within normal limits for a certain age group. Because develop-ment occurs in a sequential pattern, it is important to observe the rate of development by screening at two different points in time. Keep in mind that developmental screening is not diagnostic; its purpose is to separate children with significant developmental problems from those whose development is a variation of a normal pattern. Further evaluation is always needed when problems are found during screening. Simeonsson and Kenney point out that it is especially critical for the primary care practitioner to perform develop-mental assessments of preschool children because growth and development in this span of time is rapid, and the health care provider is often the only professional a child has contact with before entering school (13).

The Denver Developmental Screening Test (DDST) is a screening tool often used by pediatricians and nurse practitioners. It is quite useful when a developmental problem is suspected by parents or from past history or observational data. The DDST is not recommended as a regular screening tool for low risk populations due to the problem of overreferral (12). A variation of the DDST has been devised that can be given as a questionnaire to parents while waiting for their child to be seen. The Prescreening Developmental Questionnaire, as it is called, has led to some overreferrals, but has been found to be quick and economical, and has few false negatives (14). In the past, gross motor developmental milestones, such as walking and toilet training, were though to be important prognostic indicators of development. It has been found, however, that the development of speech, social and emotional development, and fine motor coordination have greater significance in terms of predictability of developmental problems (13). The DDST form is useful to have available as a reference guide of developmental norms even though one may not be administering the full test.

In addition to developmental problems, children should also be screened for behavioral disorders. These two areas are closely related, and again, there is no one tool that can screen adequately for all behavioral problems. It has been recommended that practitioners use a behavioral checklist with the parents when the child is approximately 6 months of age to increase awareness of behavioral problems. Children at risk for behavioral problems include those with chronic illnesses, such as a seizure disorder or asthma, and children whose families are undergoing stressful situations, such as divorce or movement to a new location.

INFANT FEEDING

One of the most common areas of concern for parents of new infants is what and/or how to feed their baby. Well child care visits provide an opportunity to give valuable nutritional information to parents and allow time for assessment of this area. Support and guidance given to parents in the early visits between birth and 2 months of age can help the parents' adjustment during this stressful period, and may possibly prevent common problems related to feeding, such as overfeeding and constipation. When discussing feeding with parents, try to approach the subject broadly. Parents need to receive not only information regarding adequate nutritional requirements, but also need to learn the importance of providing the food in a relaxed setting for all involved. Because of the rapid growth rate of infants—doubling birth weight by 6 months, tripling it by 12 months of age—adequate nutrition is very important for normal growth and development (15). The guidelines for feeding are relatively simple during this period and will be discussed in the following paragraphs.

BREASTFEEDING

The old adage of "breast is best" is still the preferred nutritional recommendation for young infants in the first year of life (16). The mother should be encouraged to breastfeed when possible and given much support in attempting to do so, especially during the first few weeks of her infant's life. Phone contact with health providers should be encouraged in addition to the well child visits. Family support of the mother in her attempts to breastfeed also should be encouraged. The nursing literature contains articles that are useful for those working with breastfeeding mothers (17). Breastfeeding mothers should be encouraged to get adequate fluids and rest, to try to make the feeding period relaxed, to space feeding periods (every two to three hours preferably), and to nurse from both breasts at each feeding.

Many mothers feel they should easily be able to breastfeed without problems the first few times they attempt to nurse. Inform the mother that both she and her baby are new at the process and that she should give herself time to learn slowly. Sometimes, it takes two to three weeks to establish a smooth nursing routine.

Breastfeeding has the advantage of being easily accessible. It also has been found to decrease the incidence of upper respiratory and gastrointestinal infections, and it is not allergenic (16). Its disadvantages are that it requires a healthy mother, it is associated with increased jaundice in the neonatal period, and some viral illnesses can be passed on to the baby.

One common concern of breastfeeding mothers is whether or not their infant is getting enough milk. As long as the mother's milk is coming, the baby is content after feeding and is growing adequately (gaining 3/4 to 1 ounce per day in the first six months), you can usually reassure her that the infant is getting adequate amounts. Occasionally, for various reasons, a mother will not be making or supplying adequate milk. In these instances, much encouragement and support is needed along with instructions for supplemental feedings after nursing at both breasts.

In some situations, attempts to nurse will be very frustrating for mother and infant, as well as for other family members. If the mother decides to change her infant from breast to formula, she should be helped in such a way as to alleviate feelings of guilt or failure.

Breast milk alone serves as an adequate source of nutrients for growth in the first 5 or 6 months of life, but the infant should be offered water daily in hot weather.

BOTTLE FEEDING

Infants can obtain adequate nutrition through formula feeding if it is desired or necessary. All of the standard proprietary formulas, such as Similac or

Enfamil, have the required nutrients for growth for about the first five to six months. Formula feeding has the advantages of freeing the mother's time and being more socially acceptable to some groups, and other family members can participate in feeding the baby. It has the disadvantages of expense and inconvenience (cleaning and carrying bottles, mixing formula), is a possible source of allergen, and gives no immunity to the baby. Mothers should be cautioned to read labels carefully, and mix the formula appropriately (i.e., dilute or not, as indicated). There are no firm recommendations on whether or not to sterilize bottles used for feeding young infants. It is generally thought that bottles washing in hot, soapy water from a clean water supply are adequate. Most formula ("ready to feed" and concentrated) preparations will make approximately 26 ounces to 1 quart, and should be stored in the refrigerator after opening. Any formula left in a bottle after a feeding should be discarded immediately or used in cooking for the family.

Parents should be told to avoid putting infants in bed with a bottle of formula. This could become a habit that leads to the development of severe caries in the upper incisors once the teeth have erupted. If the parents feel the baby must have a bottle to go to sleep, strongly encourage water rather than formula or juice.

Infants also can be adequately fed with formula made from evaporated milk, although in many areas this is no longer more economically advantageous than using a commercially prepared formula. Formula from evaporated milk can be made by adding 1½ cans (approximately 19 ounces) of water to 1 can of milk (13 ounces) and mixing in 2 tablespoons of corn syrup to ensure an adequate percentage of carbohydrate. No whole cow's milk (or evaporated milk mixed 1:1 with water) should be given before 7 months of age. Vitamin and iron supplements are needed when feeding with evaporated milk formula. This will be discussed in a later section.

ADDITION OF SOLIDS

There are no scientific data available that designate a specific time to introduce solids into the infant's diet. It is generally thought that a healthy full-term infant should not be given solid foods in addition to breast milk or formula until the infant is about 5 or 6 months of age (17). Because young infants do not have the motor development that enables them to either push away a spoon with their hand or turn their head away when full, it is possible to overfeed infants who are younger than 4 to 6 months. This leads not only to possible discomfort, but to possible obesity as well. Many parents feed solids to young infants thinking the infant will sleep through the night at an earlier age. There is no objective evidence to support this.

There is also no need for healthy infants less than about 4 to 6 months of age to be given nutrients other than those contained in breast milk or formula. Iron stores of full-term, healthy infants are adequate to supply them until that age without supplements.

When solids are introduced at about 5 or 6 months of age, it is generally suggested that parents start with an iron-fortified cereal to be fed with a spoon (1 to 2 tablespoons mixed with milk or formula is usually adequate). The "infant feeders" appear to lead to overfeeding and should be avoided. If iron-fortified cereal is started and given daily, any iron supplement given previously is no longer needed.

Foods to be added to the diet after cereal are usually fruits and vegetables, and generally no more than one or two new foods should be introduced per week. Cereals should be given daily until approximately 18 months of age. Partially breastfed infants should be fed foods high in protein, but this is not as necessary for older infants who are taking either formula or whole milk. By about 7 months of age, bottlefed infants should be limited to about 16 to 20 ounces of formula/milk per day. When a bottlefed infant over 6 months of age is consuming foods other than milk, including iron fortified cereals (at a level of approximately 200 grams or 1.5 jars daily), the infant can be changed to whole homogenized milk without problems (16).

Many parents are concerned about weaning at about 6 months. If an infant is taking foods other than milk, they can introduce the use of a cup at about 7 or 8 months of age. Starting at about 8 months, infants become more social and will want to use a cup like others in the family. By 1 year of age, most infants should be able to take all their liquids from a cup, provided the bottle has not been used as a pacifier. For breastfed infants, breastfeeding can continue up to 18 to 24 months, but many mothers like to wean before this time. At the ages of 9 to 10 months and again at around 15 months, infants seem to become less interested in nursing and more interested in other things in their environment. It could be suggested to mothers that these periods might be natural times to wean their infant and switch to a cup.

While discussing feeding with parents of infants of all ages, keep in mind the need for the development of sound eating habits. It should be pointed out that infants should be allowed to stop eating at the earliest sign of fullness, and that there is no benefit to feeding young infants three large meals a day instead of smaller amounts more frequently. Caution firsttime parents not to use the bottle or the breast as a pacifier; help them learn other ways to comfort and stimulate their infant. This can help avoid both obesity and dental caries while giving parents new ideas about interacting with their child.

VITAMIN AND MINERAL SUPPLEMENTATION

Vitamin and mineral supplementation is a subject of controversy. It is generally suggested that breastfed infants be given Vitamin D and iron supplements daily. Since most infant vitamin preparations contain vitamins A, C, and D and iron, this is what is usually given. Formula-fed infants do not need vitamin supplements, but may need iron supplements if formulas without iron are used. It is thought that healthy term infants, either breast or bottle fed, may not need any iron supplementation until 4 or 5 months of age when natural stores are depleted. Infants fed evaporated milk formula should be supplemented with vitamin C and iron, again, usually given in a preparation that has vitamins A and D as well. When an older infant is getting iron from foods (e.g., cereal) and needed vitamins from other sources (e.g., vegetables, fruits, and juices), supplements are no longer necessary.

A fluoride supplement of 0.25 mg daily is recommended for infants who are completely breastfed. This would not be given to infants who are drinking fluoridated water with a fluoride content of greater than 0.7 ppm. Formula-fed infants, in areas where fluoride content of water is less than 0.3 ppm, should also be given 0.25 mg/day of fluoride. To avoid oversupplementation of fluoride with resulting enamel fluorosis, young children should not be allowed to use fluoridated toothpaste until 3 years of age because they are likely to swallow the paste (16).

PARENTAL GUIDANCE

As was stated earlier, one of the objectives of well child care is to provide parents with guidance in the psychosocial aspects of child rearing, as well as anticipatory guidance in the areas of accident prevention and management of common illness. Because many young families no longer have extended families to turn to for information about child rearing, the health care provider is often the only person available to them for advice. This type of availability seems to be needed and wanted by parents, especially in the first few weeks of their infant's life. The nurse practitioner, of course, needs knowledge of normal growth and development, and cultural norms and expectations in order to give adequate guidance to parents.

Information about management of common illness and problems should be given during the early well child visits. Parents should know how to take a temperature and what temperature is considered a fever (generally over 100° F. rectally). They should be told how to manage a common cold with increased fluids, saline nose drops (1/4 teaspoon salt to 1 cup of water), and possibly a humidifier. It is generally recommended that infants less than 3 months of age with fever should be seen by a health care provider, and parents should be aware of this.

Many parents are worried about problems related to the gastrointestinal tract, including constipation, diarrhea, and spitting up. Parents should be instructed in how to give clear fluids for diarrhea or vomiting, and the difference between "spitting up" and vomiting. Constipation can usually be avoided with adequate fluid intake. Prune juice (diluted) often is used in cases of mild constipation. Dark Karo syrup (2 tablespoons to 1 quart of formula) also may be helpful. Severe or persistent constipation warrants evaluation. An enema should never be given before evaluation.

Parents usually desire information in all areas of childrearing, for example, feeding, sleeping, discipline, and toilet training. The opportunity to discuss these areas should be available at each visit, and phone contact should be encouraged when problems or concerns arise. It is generally thought that the above information should be given before problems arise, hence the term "anticipatory guidance." It is often helpful to give verbal information to parents and written material for them to have at home as a resource. Numerous books for parents with accurate, valuable information are available in paperback and are listed in the reference section.

The need to promote accident prevention cannot be overstressed. Accidents are still one of the primary causes of death and disability in children, and many can be prevented. During the newborn period, the advantages of a car seat and a safe sleeping area should be discussed. At the two month visit, warning to parents should begin on keeping small objects out of reach before the child has the skills to put things into the mouth. At the four- to six-month visit, discussions on making the home safe for crawling infants should begin. Not every parent will need or want this type of information but all should be given the opportunity to discuss these issues at each well child visit; these topics should be introduced by the nurse practitioner whether or not the parents request information. Handouts for parents can be developed by particular practitioners and are available through drug and other companies that make products for infants.

STUDY QUESTIONS

Circle all that apply.

Chris is a healthy 10 month old who has recently moved with his family to your area. This is his first visit to your clinic, and he is brought in for a check-up. His mother had his immunization record and you see that he had a DPT and oral polio (trivalent) at 8 weeks of age and again at 4 months of age. He has not received any further immunizations because of moving.

1. According to the regular schedule, what immunizations does Chris need presently?

   a. DPT and oral polio (3rd in series)
   b. DPT and oral polio (1st in new series since 6 months have elapsed since the last injection)
   c. measles, mumps, rubella (MMR)
   d. TB skin test

   Upon questioning Chris's mother about his past history, you find that he had a mild reaction to his first DPT shot (erythema at injection site, "warm in the night after the shot"), but developed a fever (104°F) after the second shot with crying, and a spell that involved "jerking" of limbs and "eyes rolling back" in his head. He was taken to the ER, but was released after his fever decreased. Although he was fussy, he seemed to do well the next day.

2. The most likely cause for his symptoms after the second series are:

   a. Severe adverse reaction to the DPT
   b. febrile seizure
   c. adverse reaction to oral polio
   d. both a and b

3. After his mother gave you this history, you tell her that:

   a. he should never have any more diphtheria, pertussis, or tetanus, because he is probably allergic to them
   b. he had a normal reaction and you will go ahead and give his immunization as planned, but he should have antipyretics concomitantly
   c. he can have DPT, but you must give it in smaller doses to avoid such severe symptoms
   d. he cannot have any more DPT, but should proceed with DT instead

4. The following signs/symptoms are fairly common side effects of DPT immunization:

   a. induration/tenderness of injection site
   b. fever (less than 104° F.)
   c. malaise
   d. screaming episodes, during which one is unable to calm the infant

Chris is brought back to you when he is 16 months old for a measles, mumps, and rubella shot. The mother was going to bring him last month but was unable to do so because of "morning sickness." She thinks she is about 2½-3 months pregnant now and does not know whether she has had rubella in the past.

5. You tell her that:

   a. Chris cannot be given his MMR because, if given the vaccine, he might expose her to rubella in her first trimester
   b. Chris should get his MMR now because the vaccine virus is not communicable and an immunized child is less likely to acquire natural rubella
   c. you will draw a rubella titer on her and immunize Chris once you know she has been exposed to rubella in the past, and thus has acquired natural immunity
   d. just wait another month to have Chris immunized because she only needs to worry about exposure during the first trimester

6. For what reason do you need to give a TB skin test before or simultaneously with the MMR vaccine?

   a. measles infection has been associated with exacerbation of quiescent tuberculosis in children
   b. A child with TB will not benefit from an MMR because of a compromised immune system, therefore the practitioner needs to be certain that the child has no active TB before giving the vaccine
   c. reaction to the MMR vaccine is worsened when the child has TB
   d. you do not need to give the TB skin test at any particular time

7. A 12-year-old boy is brought in by his mother about 30 to 40 minutes after being in a bicycle accident. His legs are badly scraped but he has no deep wounds. His mother has washed out the scrapes with running water. Your next step would be to:

   a. give him a Td booster because you assume he has probably had all of his immunizations as a child
   b. find out from the mother if he has had a primary tetanus immunization series and the approximate date of his last booster
   c. tell her that since this is not a puncture wound and she has already washed it well, her son will require no further treatment
   d. give Td booster plus 250 U Tetanus Immune Globulin (TIG)

8. You find out that his last tetanus booster was seven years previously. Therefore, you would:

   a. explain that this is a low-risk wound, therefore, he should not need a Td booster for three years
   b. give him Td now to make sure he is protected with this injury, even though the injury appears to be minor
   c. give 250 U TIG now and remind his mother that he will need a Td booster in three years
   d. give Td now, because he needs a booster every five years anyway

9. The following are contraindications for vaccination:

   a. acute, febrile illness
   b. pregnancy
   c. recent gammaglobulin or blood transfusion (within eight weeks)
   d. immunosuppressive therapy
   e. simultaneous administration of another single, live vaccine (unless they have been shown to be effective when given together)
   f. leukemia, lymphoma, or generalized malignancy

ANSWERS

1. a	6. a
2. a	7. b
3. d	8. a
4. a, b, c	9. all of the above
5. b	

SUGGESTED READING FOR PARENTS

Brazelton, T. B., *Infants and Mothers*. New York: Delacorte Press, 1969.

Caplan, F., (Ed.). *The First Twelve Months of Life*. New York: Grosset and Dunlap, 1973.

Eiger, M. S., & Olds, S. W. *The Complete Book of Breastfeeding*. New York: Bantam Books, 1972.

Leach, P. *Your Baby and Child*. New York: Alfred Knopf, 1978.

White, B. L. *The First Three Years of Life*. New York: Avon Books, 1975.

REFERENCES

1. Hoelkelman, R. A., Blatman, S., Brunnel, P. A., Friedman, S. A., & Seidel, H. M. (Eds.). *Principles of Pediatrics: Health Care of the Young.* New York: McGraw-Hill, 1978.

2. Burnip, R., Erickson, R., Barr, T. D., Shinefield, H., & Schoen, E. J. Well-child care by pediatric nurse practitioners in a large group practice. *American Journal of Diseases of Children,* 1976, *130,* 51–55.

3. Fove, H , Chamberlin, P., & Charney, E. Content and emphasis of well child visits: experienced nurse practitioners versus pediatricians. *American Journal of Diseases of Children,* 1977, *131,* 794–797.

4. Hoelkelman, R. A. What constitutes adequate well baby care? *Pediatrics,* 1975, *55,* 313–326.

5. Charney, E., and Kitzman, H. The child health nurse in private practice. *New England Journal of Medicine,* 1971, *285,* 1353–1358.

6. American Academy of Pediatrics. *Standards of Child Health Care,* 3rd ed. Evanston, Illinois, 1977.

7. Center for Disease Control. General recommendations on immunization. *Morbidity and Mortality Weekly Report,* 1976, *25, 350; 355.*

8. Committee on Infectious Diseases, *Report of the committee on infectious diseases,* 19th ed. Evanston, Illinois: American Academy of Pediatrics, 1977.

9. Center for Disease Control, Poliomyelitis prevention. *Morbidity and Mortality Weekly Report,* 1979, *28,* 510–520.

10. Center for Disease Control, measles prevention. *Morbidity and Mortality Weekly Report,* 1978, *27,* 427–437.

11. Committee on Infectious Diseases. Revised recommendations on rubella vaccine. *Pediatrics,* 1980, *65,* 1182–1184.

12. Bailey, E. N., Kiehl, P. S., Akram, D. S., Loughlin, H. H., Metcalf, T. J., Jain, R., & Perrin, J. M. Screening in pediatric practice. *Pediatric Clinics of North America, 21,* 1974, 123–165.

13. Hoelkelman, R. A., Blatman, S., Brunell, P. A., Friedman, S. A., & Seidel, H. M. (Eds.). *Principles of pediatrics: health care of the young.* New York: McGraw-Hill, 1978.

14. Ross Laboratories, *Public Health Currents,* 1976, *16.*

15. Hoelkelman, R. A., Blatman, S., Brunnell, P. A., Friedman, S. A., & Seidel, H. M. (Eds.). *op. cit.,* p. 144.

16. Fomon, S. J., Filer, L. J., Anderson, T. A., & Ziegler, E. E. Recommendations for feeding normal infants. *Pediatrics,* 1979, *63,* 52–29.

17. Grassley, J., & Davis, K. Common concerns of mothers who breastfeed. *MCN,* 1978, *3,* 347–351.

CHAPTER 4

ALLERGIC RHINITIS AND ASTHMA

Cindy S. Selleck

Allergic rhinitis and asthma affect a large number of people in the world today. Of a U.S. population of over 200 million people, 30 million suffer from allergic disorders. Of these 30 million people, it is estimated that about 5 million have asthma and 15 million have allergic rhinitis (hay fever). The remaining 10 million people include those who are afflicted with hives, eczema, headaches, and other similar allergic disorders (1).

Allergic disorders occur in people of all ages, and, although they are rarely a cause of mortality, the morbidity associated with them is great. It is estimated that 100 million days are lost from school or work each year by allergy victims (1). In school children alone, one-third of all absenteeism is thought to be due to allergic or asthmatic conditions.

This chapter focuses on the child with allergic rhinitis or asthma. Because of the prevalence, chronicity, and interrelation of these problems, it is important for the nurse practitioner to have a thorough understanding of the disease processes, their management, and the counseling necessary.

ALLERGIC RHINITIS

Allergic rhinitis, or hay fever as it is more commonly called, is the most frequent of all allergic disorders in children. Simple allergic rhinitis is caused by an allergic response to food or inhalants. In susceptible children under 6 months of age, foods (especially milk and eggs) are the most common offenders. However, in susceptible children, inhalants take on an increasing causative role from about 6 months of age on and probably account for the majority of chronic runny noses in children.

Allergic rhinitis may be seasonal (symptoms occur only during certain seasons each year) or perennial (symptoms persist for all or most of the year).

The most common seasonal inhalant offenders are the pollens. In the eastern United States, ragweed pollen is a common allergen from August through October, spring tree pollens from April through July, and summer grass pollens from May through June. The most common perennial inhalant offenders are house dust, feathers, mold spores, and animal dander, although children with perennial rhinitis are also commonly allergic to seasonal allergens as well (2).

The nose, by virtue of its placement and functions, is predisposed to frequent clinical problems. Allergic rhinitis is a disorder of the nose. The nose functions to warm, moisturize, and remove particles from inhaled air. In some people, however, because of an unknown predisposition, inhalation of certain particles causes an antigen-antibody interaction that results in an allergic response. In allergic rhinitis, the allergic response is localized to the site of entry of the offending inhaled particles (antigens). In other words, the antigen-antibody reaction and subsequent symptoms take place within the respiratory tract. The allergic reaction causes cellular damage of specific sensitized cells (mast cells) within the nasal and respiratory mucosa, which results in the release of histamine and other vasoactive enzymes from these cells. It is these enzymes that initiate a local inflammatory response and cause the excessive mucus secretion and vasoconstriction of nasal and respiratory mucosa that are so characteristic of allergic rhinitis.

HISTORY

The child with allergic rhinitis typically appears with a history of sneezing, itching, runny and stuffy nose, red, itching eyes, burning and itching throat, malaise, and possibly complaints of itchy, stuffy ears. Children with allergic rhinitis frequently rub their noses in a characteristic manner: with the palm of their hand pushing the tip of the nose upward. This rubbing has been termed the "allergic salute" and tends to produce what is known as the "allergic crease" across the child's nose.

Also typical in these children is a bluish discoloration under both eyes known as "allergic shiners," caused by venous stasis resulting from interference with blood flow through the edematous nasal mucosa. Because nasal mucosa becomes so edematous in allergic rhinitis and these children often are unable to breathe through their noses, they become mouth breathers with the characteristic gaping mouths. Snoring and restlessness during sleep also results from not being able to breathe through their noses.

Not surprisingly, allergic children often are oblivious to their own symptoms. Parents may be the first to notice their child's chronic or intermittent sneezing, sniffling, and runny nose. Or they may complain that the child makes all sorts of unpleasant noises by constantly sniffing, snorting, or clearing the throat. They also may notice the child's increased fatigue and the interference with rest that allergic rhinitis symptoms can cause. If the rhinitis is seasonal, the child is normally free from symptoms between the offending seasons. But, if the rhinitis is perennial, the child can be plagued by symptoms throughout the year, becoming particularly severe during the typical offending seasons.

PHYSICAL EXAMINATION

Physical examination of the child with uncomplicated allergic rhinitis generally shows the same typical changes regardless of the cause. Mucosa of the nose, throat, and soft palate usually appears pale or bluish-grey, shiny, and swollen, and a thin, watery or mucus-like nasal discharge may be present. Nasal polyps may be evident, especially in the child with perennial rhinitis who has chronic nasal irritation. The uvula and tonsils become pale, greyish, and swollen. The pale color of the uvula and soft palate is an important differentiating factor between an allergic and infectious cause of the symptoms. When the nose and throat are infected, the uvula and soft palate generally have an erythematous, or reddened appearance (1).

On examination of the child's eyes, a mild, bilateral conjunctivitis may be apparent, as well as mild periorbital edema and allergic shiners. An allergic crease may be evident horizontally across the lower portion of the child's nose.

Uncomplicated allergic rhinitis causes no symptoms of the lower respiratory tract. Therefore, examination of the child's chest and auscultation of lung fields should be completely normal.

The clinical manifestations of allergic rhinitis cause these children to be more susceptible to certain other disorders. The edematous nasal and respiratory mucosa is more susceptible to invading, infectious organisms. Therefore, children with allergic rhinitis are at greater risk for colds and other respiratory tract infections. Because of the edematous nasal and oral mucosa, with possible subsequent blockage of sinuses or eustachian tubes, these children also are prone to sinusitis and serous otitis media. Because one-third or more of all children with allergic rhinitis may develop asthma, it is important for the nurse practitioner to be alert to the development of cough and wheezing, signs that can signal the onset of asthma.

DIAGNOSTIC TESTS

A thorough history and a physical examination are helpful and necessary procedures in the evaluation of a child who appears with symptoms of allergic rhinitis. Because there is a relative increase in eosinophils in association with antigen-antibody reactions, a nasal smear to look for the percentage of eosinophils can be helpful in the diagnosis of allergic rhinitis. This can be done by using a cotton-tipped applicator to obtain some nasal discharge, spreading the discharge on a glass slide, and staining it. More than 3 to 4% eosinophils suggests an allergic problem (3).

MANAGEMENT

Since children with successfully treated allergic rhinitis are much less likely to develop asthma, the goals for managing allergic rhinitis in the child are allergen avoidance and alleviation of symptoms. It cannot be overemphasized that a thorough and detailed history is by far the most helpful tool to the nurse practitioner in managing the child with allergic rhinitis. A careful family history is also important since allergic rhinitis is often a hereditary condition. If identification of the offending antigens can be made by history, steps can be taken to avoid contact with these antigens. It may be impossible to completely avoid all identified allergens, but it usually is feasible to minimize contact, thereby reducing the incidence and severity of subsequent allergic reactions (4).

Counseling

If the allergic rhinitis is seasonal, a knowledge of which pollens are present during various times of the year in that particular location will help the nurse practitioner to determine the probable cause of the symptoms. Counseling the child and parents about avoiding areas heavily concentrated with ragweed, trees, or grasses during the pollinating seasons, and sleeping with bedroom windows closed or with an air conditioner on may be especially helpful.

For those children with perennial allergic rhinitis, environmental control of common allergens is beneficial. Parents should be instructed on how to create a dust-free bedroom for their allergic child, and the child should be counseled about avoiding plant products (kapok, cotton), animal products (feathers, horse hair, wool, fur), animals and damp places, such as basements, where molds frequently thrive.

Pharmacology

Drug therapy using oral antihistamines, oral antihistamine-decongestant combinations, and topical decongestant nasal sprays or drops is appropriate for symptomatic treatment of allergic rhinitis.

Antihistamines. Antihistamines are the most widely used and effective remedies for allergic rhinitis. They act by competing with histamine for receptor sites. This antihistamine effect causes a decrease in the amount of mucus secretion, thereby relieving the rhinorrhea. Because antihistamines do not antagonize histamine that has already been released, but rather prevent further release, they are most effective if taken continuously for a period of days or weeks rather than intermittently during symptomatic periods.

Antihistamines may cause drowsiness although the degree of sedation varies between the different preparations. Anticholinergic side effects, such as dry mouth, blurred vision, urinary retention, and constipation may be associated with high doses. If antihistamines are taken regularly for several weeks or months, there is a tendency to develop a tolerance to them, evidenced by decreased effectiveness. If this occurs, switching to a different antihistamine usually corrects the problem. Antihistamine preparations are available both as nonprescription and prescription medications.

Decongestants. Decongestants are sympathomimetic amines and are used either alone or in combination with an antihistamine to relieve nasal stuffiness associated with allergic rhinitis. The decongestant, given orally or as nasal spray or drops, causes constriction of the dilated arterioles within the nasal mucosa thereby temporarily reducing blood flow and causing shrinkage of the swollen mucous membranes.

If label directions are followed, topical decongestant application provides prompt relief of nasal congestion. Chronic use or overuse of decongestant nasal spray or drops, however, causes a rebound phenomenon with worsening nasal congestion and edema. Oral decongestants have the advantage of a longer duration of action and no rebound congestion, although the degree of decongestant relief is not as great as with the topical preparations. Side effects of oral decongestants include tachycardia, increased blood pressure, and nervousness. Decongestant preparations are available both as nonprescription and prescription medications.

Hyposensitization. Hyposensitization, or immunotherapy, may be necessary in those children whose allergic rhinitis symptoms are not adequately relieved by both contact avoidance and use of antihistamines and decongestants. Those children with perennial, year-round symptoms and those whose seasonal symptoms are severe are good candidates for hyposensitization or "allergy shots."

After a series of skin tests to determine what substances the child is allergic to, hyposensitization consists of frequent, subcutaneous injections of increasing amounts of these allergens. A top dose, the amount that induces a state of hyporeactivity, is reached and this is injected as a maintenance dose at frequent intervals (4). The idea behind hyposensitization is to make the allergic child less sensitive to his or her allergens.

Referral

Although nurse practitioners do not perform hyposensitization therapy, it is important for them to be aware of the benefit this therapy can provide to certain children. In cases of significant allergic rhinitis symptoms, despite appropriate environmental control and pharmacologic management, the nurse practitioner should initiate referral to an allergist for appropriate hyposensitization therapy.

ASTHMA

Bronchial asthma is a major cause of both acute and chronic illnesses in children. It accounts for approximately 25% of all school days lost and 33% of all chronic conditions during childhood (5). In children, the onset of asthma is most common during the first five years of life, and it occurs twice as frequently in boys until adolescence, when the sex ratio begins to equalize.

Asthma is a disease of the airways that is characterized by an increased responsiveness or hyperactivity of the tracheobronchial tree to a variety of stimuli (6). The major pathophysiologic changes that occur with asthma are recurrent, reversible bronchospasm with narrowing of the airways, edema of the bronchial mucosa, and increased secretion of bronchial mucus. The factors that can cause these changes to occur are numerous. In fact, the airways of children with asthma have been shown to become hyperresponsive to a multiplicity of stimuli, including smoke, fumes, pollutions, exercise, foods, drugs, changes in temperature and barometric pressure, respiratory tract infections, emotional upsets, as well as the typical allergic rhinitis offenders (pollens, house dust, feathers, mold, and animal dander). If one or more factors can be identified as the inciting agent of an asthma attack, the disease is termed extrinsic or allergic asthma. But if the inciting agent is unknown, the asthma is called intrinsic or idiosyncratic. In children, extrinsic asthma is the type most commonly seen and frequently is associated with a personal or family history of other allergic disorders, such as allergic rhinitis or eczema.

HISTORY

Asthma is an episodic disease in which acute episodes alternate with symptom-free periods. The severity of symptoms a child experiences with an acute episode depends on the amount of airway obstruction that is present. For the most part, as obstruction increases, so do the number and intensity of symptoms. Episodes typically begin abruptly with a nonproductive cough frequently a presenting symptom, followed by dyspnea, chest tightness, and prolonged expirations. Wheezing is usually prominent and may be heard both during inspiration and expiration. The child typically becomes anxious and apprehensive as breathing becomes more difficult.

For some as yet unexplained reason, asthma attacks often occur during the middle of the night. Generally, acute episodes are shortlived, lasting from a few minutes to hours. Because the lung changes that occur with asthma are considered largely reversible, most children completely recover and are symptom-free after an acute attack. A few asthmatic children, however, seem to experience a mild degree of airway obstruction continuously (6).

PHYSICAL EXAMINATION

A thorough history and physical examination are extremely important parts of the assessment and management of the asthmatic child. Between acute episodes, when the child is normally symptom-free, the physical examination is usually normal also. Height and weight, however, should be routinely measured and recorded on serial graphs in the chart because growth delay may occur secondary to uncontrolled reversible bronchospasm. Deviation from established normal growth patterns can be one of the first signs of asthma during infancy and childhood (5). Should this be apparent, consultation with or referral to a physician would be indicated.

Other signs that may be seen in asymptomatic asthmatic children are nasal polyps, particularly if the child has extrinsic asthma associated with typical allergic rhinitis symptoms. Coughing, prolonged expiration, and rhonchi following strenuous exercise, which are indicative of ongoing obstructive airway disease, may be noted. An increased anterior-posterior chest diameter may be seen in children with more chronic, severe disease (5).

During acute asthmatic episodes, both the appearance and physical examination of the asthmatic child are striking. Respiratory rate is rapid, usually more than 24 respirations per minute, and there is prolonged expiration with expiratory wheezing and often inspiratory wheezing that can be heard without the aid of a stethoscope. Because of air trapped within the lungs, percussion over lung fields is hyperresonant. Use of accessory neck and intercostal muscles with subsequent intercostal retractions may be apparent. Cyanosis of lips and nail beds may occur with severely compromised lung function. Perspiration and fatigue generally occur as the child expends more energy to breathe. Depending on the etiology of the episode, fever or nasal congestion and rhinorrhea may be evident.

DIAGNOSTIC TESTS

There is no single laboratory test that is conclusive for asthma. Rather, the history and physical examination findings, along with the results from various laboratory tests confirm the diagnosis initially.

Laboratory tests that may be helpful in the asthmatic child include a nasal, sputum, or blood smear to look for eosinophils; during acute episodes of extrinsic asthma, increased numbers of eosinophils can be found in nasal secretions, sputum, and peripheral blood. These tests will be normal between attacks. Skin testing to identify allergens may be helpful in the child with extrinsic asthma. Or, if allergens are suspected as the inciting factor, provocative challenge tests with the suspected offending food or inhalant will show clinical reactions in a positive test. If specific allergens are identified, the child will benefit from contact avoidance and possibly hyposensitization.

If it is the child's first visit with a complaint or suspicion of asthma, a baseline chest roentgenogram is usually indicated to help rule out other childhood conditions that might cause wheezing. Chest x ray films taken during an acute asthma episode will show bilateral hyperinflation and bronchial thickening. After the initial diagnosis, chest roentgenograms are generally not indicated during acute episodes unless the attacks are accompanied by unusual symptoms, persistent fever, or are unresponsive to standard therapy (5).

Pulmonary function studies are indicated periodically in asthmatic children to monitor lung function. Generally, children 6 years old and older can cooperate enough to perform routine spirometry, including forced vital capacity (FVC), forced expiratory volume in one second (FEV_1), maximal midexpiratory flow rate (MMFR), and functional residual capacity (FRC). Vital capacity, the amount of air that can be forcefully expired after a maximal inspiration, is usually normal in asthmatic children, although the FEV_1, and MMFR are below normal and the FRC is increased. These serial measurements of lung function are necessary in order to adjust drug therapy for restoring and maintaining lung function in the asthmatic child (5).

MANAGEMENT

Although asthma cannot be cured and children do not outgrow it, good control of asthma is possible and many children do have fewer acute attacks as they grow older. The nurse practitioner may have the major role in educating the child and family about the disease, in making sure all recommendations are fully understood, and in monitoring the child periodically. The nurse practitioner may be in the best position to pick up problems the child or family may be experiencing with the disease, and to provide necessary support and counseling. With appropriate management by both the nurse practitioner and physician, childhood asthma can be well controlled, normal lung function maintained, and most children can lead normal lives.

Counseling

Obtaining a thorough and detailed history, including a family history, is particularly important in managing the asthmatic child. If extrinsic asthma is determined by history, skin testing, or provocative challenge tests, the nurse practitioner should first counsel the child and parents on how to institute environmental controls. The same environmental controls that are recommended for allergic rhinitis also hold true for asthma (maintaining a dust-free bedroom, avoiding plant and animal products, animals, damp, moldy places, and pollens). If avoidance of allergens is successful, the frequency of acute attacks should be significantly reduced. Hyposensitization injections are also so frequently helpful in desensitizing the child to his or her offending allergens, thereby reducing the number of acute asthma episodes.

The effect asthma can have on a child and family is devastating at times. The child may experience delays in psychological, physical, and educational development and the disease may significantly disrupt the family's emotional and financial security (5). For these reasons, counseling and education of the asthmatic child and family are of prime importance.

Pharmacology

Pharmacologic therapy is an important part of asthma management in the child. Drug therapy may be needed only when the child experiences acute episodes if the disease is mild and episodes are infrequent. If the child has frequent, more severe attacks, however, constant prophylactic pharmacologic therapy may be indicated. The nurse practitioner should consult with a physician about appropriate drug therapy before initiating any medications.

Bronchodilators. Bronchodilating drugs, especially the methylxanthines such as theophylline and the sympathomimetic amines (beta-adrenergic agents), such as ephedrine and epinephrine, are mainstays of asthma therapy. Short- or long-acting oral theophylline is often used prophylactically and in the symptomatic relief of bronchospasm associated with bronchial asthma. Theophylline works through relaxation of smooth muscle and bronchiolar tone. Its main side effects are nausea, vomiting, and anorexia. The sympathomimetic amines are more potent bronchodilators. Ephedrine is effective orally in causing bronchodilation, and, because it has a slow onset and long duration of action, it is used to prevent attacks in children with mild to moderate disease. Epinephrine, effective only parenterally or via inhalation, is used in severe episodes or in status asthmaticus to relieve acute bronchospasm. Epinephrine is contained in all nonprescription aerosol products marketed for relief of asthma. The major side effects of the sympathomimetic agents are nervousness, restlessness, palpitations, and tremor. Chronic use of these drugs leads to tolerance.

Cromolyn Sodium. Cromolyn sodium (Intal) acts prophylactically to prevent bronchospasm. It is a topical agent that prevents release of histamine. Cromolyn comes in powder-filled capsules that are pierced and inhaled through a spinhaler. It is most effective in children with extrinsic asthma and has been shown to decrease the need for both bronchodilators and cortico-steroids in these children.

Corticosteroids. Corticosteroids are potent drugs and should be reserved for those children whose chronic, severe asthma cannot be controlled by other drugs alone. Prednisone is the steroid most commonly used in the treatment of asthma. Steroids are best used short-term (no more than ten days), although if long-term therapy is necessary, an alternate day schedule should be used. Side effects of steroids include fluid retention, increased appetite, weight gain, and growth retardation.

Vanceril. Vanceril (beclomethasone dipropionate), a synthetic cortico-steroid supplied as an aerosol powder, has not been shown to produce the side effects seen with steroids. It is particularly effective in those children with steroid-dependent asthma; it often allows steroid therapy to be reduced or completely discontinued. Side effects of Vanceril include dry mouth, cough, and oral candidiasis.

Referral

The goal of managing childhood asthma is to try to maintain adequate lung function so that these children can lead normally active lives with minimal interference from lung dysfunction. As stated previously, the nurse practitioner's major concern is to educate the child and family about the disease, to make sure all recommendations are fully understood, and to monitor the child periodically. The initiation of medication is primarily the role of the physician. If hyposensitivity is necessary, the physician and nurse practitioner may refer the child to an allergist.

STUDY QUESTIONS

Circle all that apply.

Seven-year-old Jimmy is in your clinic today because his mother complains that he sniffs and snorts all the time and she is sure there must be something wrong with him. From your history, you find that Jimmy has a chronic runny nose and that he always seems to be rubbing his eyes. Although Jimmy's symptoms persist year-round, they seem to be worse during the spring and early summer. There is a positive family history of hay fever and Jimmy's mother reports that he had eczema as an infant.

1. On physical examination of Jimmy you note mild bilateral conjunctivitis and pale, swollen nasal mucosa. What other signs might you expect to find?

    a. nasal polyps
    b. allergic shiners
    c. bilateral expiratory wheezing
    d. erythematous mucosa of pharynx and soft palate

2. From your history and physical examination you determine that Jimmy has:

    a. seasonal allergic rhinitis
    b. bronchial asthma
    c. perennial allergic rhinitis
    d. streptococcal pharyngitis

3. Which of the following diagnostic tests are appropriate with Jimmy?

    a. throat culture
    b. nasal smear
    c. routine spirometry
    d. chest x-ray film

4. You determine that Jimmy has perennial allergic rhinitis. Which of the following would you include in your plan of management?

    a. counseling Jimmy and his mother on instituting environmental controls
    b. suggesting to Jimmy's mother that she buy him a dog, because a pet would be particularly helpful to him at this point in his life
    c. starting Jimmy on daily therapy with Chlor-Trimeton
    d. referring Jimmy to an allergist for hyposensitization if constant avoidance and antihistamines do not significantly reduce symptoms

5. Jimmy's mother brings him back to the clinic two months later. She says he has been taking the Chlor-Trimeton daily as instructed and although he seemed much improved for the first six weeks, his nose has begun to run daily again and he sniffs and snorts like before. You decide to:

    a. refer Jimmy to a physician because of unresponsive symptoms
    b. review environmental controls with Jimmy and his mother again to determine if they fully understand and are adhering to your recommendations
    c. add Dimetapp Extentabs, an antihistamine-decongestant combination, reassuring Jimmy and his mother that the Chlor-Trimeton alone was not enough medication

d. stop the Chlor-Trimeton and begin Dimetapp Extentabs, reassuring Jimmy and his mother that developing tolerance to antihistamines is not uncommon.

Five-year-old Beth has had asthma for four years. It was first detected during an episode of bronchiolitis when she was an infant. She is currently maintained on 50 mg theophylline po q6h. Her father brings her into the clinic today for her routine immunizations.

6. On history, you find that although Beth takes her theophylline regularly, cold weather and vigorous exercise seem to trigger episodes of wheezing and shortness of breath. You know that when one or more factors can be identified as the inciting agent of an asthma attack, the disease is termed:

   a. intrinsic asthma
   b. extrinsic asthma

7. Which of the following would you want to be sure to include in your examination of Beth today?

   a. chest roentgenogram
   b. pulmonary function studies
   c. height and weight
   d. blood test for eosinophilia

8. On examination of her chest, you note that Beth has mild, bilateral, expiratory wheezing. You consult with your preceptor and jointly decide to increase her daily dose of theophylline. You see Beth for a follow-up visit three days later and, although her physical examination is normal, her father states she has been nauseous and has vomited three times during the past 24 hours. You decide to:

   a. assure her father that Beth probably has a viral gastroenteritis and recommend dietary modifications until her symptoms subside
   b. draw a theophylline level
   c. counsel Beth and her father on expected side effects of drug therapy for asthma
   d. discontinue the theophylline

9. You and your preceptor decide to place Beth on 50 mg theophylline po q6h and 20 mg Cromolyn Sodium (Intal) qid. You know that the following are true about cromolyn sodium:

   a. it is most effective in children with extrinsic asthma
   b. it is relatively inexpensive
   c. it works topically to prevent release of histamine

d. it may help to decrease the need for both bronchodilators and corticosteroids

10. Beth's father expresses concern about his daughter's asthma. In counseling her father about the disease, which would be the best advice?

a. Beth is essentially an invalid and her activities should be severely
restricted
b. in all likelihood, Beth will outgrow her asthma
c. Beth is likely to develop chronic obstructive pulmonary disease as
she gets older
d. with appropriate management, Beth's asthma can be well controlled,
normal lung function maintained, and Beth can lead a normal life

ANSWERS

1. a, b   6. b
2. c   7. c
3. b   8. b
4. a, c, d   9. a, c, d
5. b, d   10. d

REFERENCES

1. Swineford, O. *Asthma and hay fever.* Springfield, IL.: Charles C. Thomas, 1973.
2. Hoole, A. J., Greenberg, R. A., & Pichard, C. G. *Patient care guidelines for family nurse practitioners.* Boston: Little, Brown, 1976.
3. Capell, P. T., & Case, D. B. *Ambulatory care manual for nurse practitioners.* Philadelphia: J. B. Lippincott, 1976
4. Kempe, C. H., Silver, H. K., & O'Brien, D. *Current pediatric diagnosis and treatment.* Los Angeles: Lange Medical Publications, 1978.
5. Gershwin, M. E. *Bronchial asthma, principles of diagnosis and treatment.* New York: Grune and Stratton, 1981.
6. Thorn, G. W. et al. *Harrison's principles of internal medicine.* New York: McGraw-Hill, 1977.

CHAPTER **5**

UPPER RESPIRATORY INFECTIONS

Terry E. Tippett Neilson

The pediatric client frequently presents with problems of the upper respiratory tract. These include external otitis, acute otitis media, acute sinusitis, and pharyngitis. Common viral illnesses with respiratory tract components are also common complaints, for example, mononucleosis and influenza.

EXTERNAL OTITIS

External otitis is an inflammatory process of the skin and glands of the external ear canal. Although it can occur spontaneously, it is more likely the result of abrasion to the canal's skin by bobby pins, tooth picks, paper clips, or cotton-tipped applicators. These objects can remove the canal's protective layer of wax and injure the skin, leaving it vulnerable to secondary infections. The bacteria that frequently invade the injured skin is a mixed infection including *Pseudomonas, Proteus,* and *Staphylococcus aureus.*

HISTORY

The pain of external otitis varies from annoying itch to a severe continuous ear pain. The pain is aggravated by moving the pinna. Frequently, the child notices a purulent discharge from the affected ear. Often there is a history of swimming before the onset of ear pain. The bacteria from the water are allowed to invade the unprotected injured skin of the canal and proliferate.

PHYSICAL EXAMINATION

Either pressure to the tragus or moving the pinna will produce pain. Since the infection is localized to the superficial skin, inspection usually reveals an edematous, red canal that is often filled with a purulent discharge.

DIAGNOSTIC TESTS

Usually one will not culture the external ear canal unless it is unresponsive to therapy. If a culture is indicated, the following mediums are used:

1. Blood agar—*pneumococcus, Streptococcus, Staphylococcus*
2. Chocolate agar—*Hemophilus influenzae*
3. Eosin methylene blue (EMB)—*E. coli, Klebsiella, Proteus, Pseudomonas*

MANAGEMENT

Since external otitis is usually a superficial bacterial infection of the skin, topical antibiotics play a significant part in its management. To reduce the number of future infections, parent education is essential.

Counseling

The goal of counseling is to prevent future infections. Stress to the child and parents that the cause of the initial infection probably is due to trauma caused by attempts to clean the ear. Furthermore, parents and child should be educated to keep ears dry by allowing water to drain from them after bathing or swimming. Cotton-tipped applicators should not be used. People who are predisposed to external otitis should be encouraged to wear ear plugs while swimming.

Pharmacology

Since external otitis usually involves only the superficial layer of the canal's skin, treatment is local. Topical antibiotic otic drugs commonly used are those containing polymyxin and neomycin with hydrocortisone (used to reduce inflammation). The treatment period is two weeks.

Referral

An otologic referral is necessary when cartilage in the ear canal is visible, in an unstable diabetic child, or if the external otitis is unresponsive to therapy.

ACUTE OTITIS MEDIA

Acute otitis media is a suppurative infection of the middle ear. Two-thirds of all children will have one attack of otitis by the time they are 8 years of age. However, it occurs most frequently in children under 2 years of age because of the straight angle of their eustachian tube. This allows the easy spread of microorganisms from an infected nasopharynx to the normally sterile middle ear space.

Following a single episode of acute otitis media, an effusion may persist in the middle ear for up to several months. This condition is known as serous otitis media and is a common cause of temporary hearing loss.

Although some cases of otitis media are viral in origin, the following are the common bacterial agents.

Birth to three months
1. *Escherichia coli*
2. *Klebsiella pneumoniae*
3. *Staphylococcus aureus*

Three months to eight years
1. *Hemophilus influenzae* accounts for about 33% of cases in infancy, but becomes less frequent with increasing age.
2. *Diplococcus pneumoniae* is responsible for greater than 50% of the cases.
3. *Streptococcus* and *Staphylococcus* are found in fewer than 5% of patients.

Eight years and older
1. *D. pneumoniae* accounts for the majority of the cases in the older patient.
2. *H. influenzae* is being found more frequently in older children. The overall incidence is low.

HISTORY

The initial complaint is often a constant or intermittent ear pain that may radiate over the involved side of the head. Infants and toddlers may pull at the affected ear. Usually accompanying the earache is a feeling of fullness and impaired hearing. Frequently, these symptoms occur within a few days after the onset of a viral upper respiratory infection. Fever, irritability, and nonspecific gastrointestinal symptoms (anorexia, vomiting, and diarrhea) are commonly reported.

If the tympanic membrane ruptures, the child will often report a spontaneous disappearance of pain. Purulent secretions from the middle ear space can drain into the external ear causing an external otitis.

PHYSICAL EXAMINATION

To diagnose an acute otitis media, one must be able to inspect the tympanic membrane. This can be a difficult task if wax is blocking the view or the child is uncooperative. It is necessary to remove any cerumen or dry skin to properly inspect the tympanic membrane. Classically, acute otitis media appears as a red, bulging tympanic membrane that has lost its landmarks. However, in its early stages, hyperemia may be the only sign. Since a healthy, crying child also has red tympanic membranes, it is important to be able to distinguish between the two. Loss of mobility of the tympanic membrane is the key to acute otitis media. To test for mobility, one uses pneumatic otoscopy.

Conductive hearing loss can be evaluated by the Weber and Rinne tests. The Weber will show laterality in the affected ear, while the Rinne will show bone conduction better than air conduction in the affected ear.

DIAGNOSTIC TEST

Usually it is not necessary to culture the middle ear unless it is unresponsive to therapy. If a culture is indicated, needle aspiration or a myringotomy will be performed and the following medium are used:
1. Blood agar—*Pneumococcus, Streptococcus, Staphylococcus*
2. Chocolate agar—*Hemophilus influenzae*
3. Eosin methylene blue (EMB)—*E. coli, Klebsiella, Proteus, Pseudomonas*

MANAGEMENT

Antibiotics play a major role in the management of otitis media in children. Parent education is important to reduce the number of future middle ear infections.

Counseling

To reduce the incidence of future attacks, the parents need to have a sound understanding of the pathology and management involved in otitis media. Educating the parents on the following information is essential:

1. The position and anatomy of eustachian tube is the reason that young children have a higher incidence of acute otitis media.
2. Elevating an infant and young child during feeding is believed to decrease the incidence of otitis media. The parents should be encouraged not to give their child a bottle of milk at bedtime.
3. After a single bout of acute otitis media, the child may have decreased hearing in the affected ear for as long as 10 weeks.
4. Educating the parents on the importance of continuing the full 10-day course of antibiotics.
5. Finally, explaining the importance of follow-up visits.

Pharmacology

During the first few days of the infection, antihistamines and decongestants are frequently prescribed to keep down the mucous production. However, the effectiveness of their use in facilitating drainage of fluid from the middle ear by keeping the eustachian tube patent is the subject of controversy.

The microorganisms vary with the age of the patient. The nurse practitioner needs to select the appropriate chemotherapy agent.

Birth to Three Months. The nurse practitioner refers the infant or consults on therapy. The academic approach for treating very young infants is needle aspiration of the middle ear fluid or myringotomy for culture and antibiotic sensitivity testing. The rationale is that this is a potentially serious systemic infection with the risk of gram-negative septicemia.

Three Months to Eight Years. Since *H. influenzae* has an increased risk as the cause for otitis media in this age group, but not exclusively, a broad spectrum antibiotics should be used.

1. Ampicillin is frequently used because of its effectiveness against *H. influenza*. Also, it is the least expensive of all antibiotics used for otitis media. However, there are many disadvantages:
   a. Its absorption is affected by the gastric acid and gastric contents, therefore, it needs to be administered one hour before meals.
   b. Dosage schedule is four times a day.
   c. Common side effects are diarrhea (especially over 1 gram daily doses) and skin rashes.
   d. There are increasing incidences of resistant strains of microorganisms to ampicillin.
2. Amoxicillin has been shown to have identical antimicrobial activity for otitis media as ampicillin. Other advantages of amoxicillin are:

    a. Its absorption is unaffected by gastric acid or gastric contents, there-
fore, it can be given with meals.

    b. It has a more rapid absorption from the gastrointestinal tract, there-
fore, causing fewer upsets.

    c. It has a less frequent dosage schedule which might increase patient
compliance.

    d. There are very few resistant strains of microorganisms to amoxicillin.
The main disadvantage of amoxicillin is that it costs between 25 to
50% more than ampicillin. When treating patients with limited financial resources, the cost should be taken into consideration.

3. Trimethoprim-sulfamethoxazole has been shown to be as effective as the
other drugs previously discussed for the first line of treatment against the
microorganisms of otitis media. Other advantages of trimethoprim-sulfamethoxazole are:

    a. Since this drug is not a penicillin analog, it is often used when allergies
to penicillin are suspected.

    b. The dosage schedule is only twice daily, therefore, compliance might
be improved.

    The main disadvantage of trimethoprim-sulfamethoxazole is that it costs
twice as much as ampicillin. Many clients may be unable to afford treatment.
Even in prepaid systems, cost control is important and liberal dispensing of
this drug is often discouraged.

4. Erythromycin ethylsuccinate and sulfisoxazole have the following advantages:

    a. Since they are not penicillin analogs, they are often used when allergy
to penicillin is known.

    b. They are active against some *H. influenzae* strains that are known to
be ampicillin-resistant.

    The disadvantages to erythromycin ethylsuccinate and sulfisoxazole are:

    a. There are some *H. influenzae* resistant strains to these drugs.

    b. Since there are two drugs involved, compliance may be a problem.
There is a commercial product that combines these two drugs, however, the cost is about twice as much as ampicillin.

Eight Years and Older.   Since *D. pneumoniae* accounts for the majority of
cases in the older client, penicillin is the preferred medication. If known
allergy to penicillin exists, erythromycin would be the drug of choice.

Referral

Referral is indicated in the following situations:

1. Fever, drainage, and pain persist longer than 48 hours after antibiotic therapy has been initiated.
2. The patient has three or more recurrent episodes of acute otitis media during the otitis season.
3. Conductive hearing loss or serous otitis persists longer than six weeks.
4. If there are signs of mastoiditis (swelling over the mastoid process, or displacement of the external ear laterally and inferiorly).

ACUTE PHARYNGITIS

Acute pharyngitis is an infection of the mucous membranes of the pharynx, adenoids, or tonsils. As its name implies, acute tonsillitis is an infection of the tonsils. However, there are no significant differences in the clinical presentation or management between the two entities.

The majority of sore throats are viral. The more common types of bacteria that are capable of producing pharyngitis are *Hemophilus influenzae,* *Pneumococcus,* and *Streptococcus* (Groups A, B, C, D). Group A beta-hemolytic streptococci is the only one that requires antibiotic intervention.

Bacterial pharyngitis, as compared to viral, has a more abrupt onset, produces a more severe systemic illness, has a longer duration, and is associated with more severe complications. Unfortunately, atypical presentations of both are frequent, making it virtually impossible to distinguish between the two on clinical findings alone. Therefore, the only reliable method of differentiating between a viral sore throat and a bacterial one is by a throat culture.

As stated above, group A beta-hemolytic streptococci is the only common pathogen of the pharynx that requires antibiotics. This antibiotic therapy does not shorten the length of the illness, nor does it make any of the clinical symptoms less severe. However, if antibiotic therapy is begun within nine days after the onset of the infection, it does prevent the rheumatic fever sequelae. Unfortunately, it does not prevent acute glomerulonephritis.

HISTORY

Many clinical studies indicate that children with viral sore throats are more likely to complain of a gradual onset, rhinorrhea, headache, mild hoarseness, and a low-grade fever. On the other hand, bacterial infections are more often responsible for complaints of an abrupt onset, dysphagia, arthralgias, myalgias, malaise, and fever greater than 101°F.

PHYSICAL EXAMINATION

Similar to the history, the physical findings vary greatly. Inspection of the mucous membranes of the throat may reveal a mild to severe hyperemia with or without enlarged, erythematous tonsils with exudate. Nasal discharge varies from thin watery to purulent. Cervical lymphadenopathy may be present. Clinical studies indicate that streptococcal infections are more commonly associated with enlarged erythematous tonsils with exudate, purulent nasal discharge, and cervical lymphadenopathy.

DIAGNOSTIC TESTS

Although studies associate different clinical findings with viral and bacterial infections, atypical presentations of each are very common. It is extremely difficult to distinguish between the two on the basis of clinical findings alone. A more reliable method is by performing a throat culture.

On the blood agar media, hemolytic streptococcal colonies are encircled by a zone of hemolysis. To differentiate between a group A and a nongroup A beta-hemolytic streptococcal growth, place a bacitracin disk on the blood agar. The group A growth will be inhibited by the bacitracin disk. It is important to point out that throat cultures are not entirely accurate. Unfortunately, they are responsible for about 10% false-negative and 20% false-positive results.

MANAGEMENT

Since the majority of sore throats are viral, medication plays a minor role in the treatment. Parent education is the cornerstone of managing a child with pharyngitis.

Counseling

Many parents are convinced that a sore throat requires an antibiotic. Unless the nurse practitioner takes the time to explain why antibiotics are only useful against the group A beta-hemolytic streptococal throat infections, the parents are likely to leave the office unhappy. The parents need to have a sound understanding of the disease process and the management of a group A beta-hemolytic streptococcal infection and one that is not.

The nurse practitioner should advise all sore throat clients on the following supportive and symptomatic care:

1. Encourage rest.
2. Gargle with warm salt water.
3. Eat a well-balanced diet and increase oral fluid intake.
4. Humidify air to soothe the irritated throat and keep membranes moist. Basins of water may be placed around the house, a vaporizer may be used, or steam from a sink or shower may be inhaled.

Pharmacology

To control fever and myalgia, analgesics and antipyretics are prescribed. Compounds containing aspirin or acetaminophen are used.

Antibiotics are reserved for those children with a positive throat culture. However, if the nurse practitioner has a high suspicion of a streptococcal pharyngitis and is concerned that the child will not be seen again, advance treatment with antibiotics is appropriate. Oral or intramuscular (Bicillin) penicillin are drugs of choice. If there is a known penicillin allergy, erythromycin is the preferred medication.

REFERRAL

If a child misses more than two days of school each month because of repeated episodes of tonsillitis, a tonsillectomy may be indicated.

Referral to a physician is recommended for those children with a peritonsillar abscess, epiglottitis, or sore throat symptoms still present after three weeks.

INFECTIOUS MONONUCLEOSIS

There is much to learn about this common infectious disease of late adolescence and young adulthood. It is believed to be caused by the Epstein-Barr virus (EBv), a member of the herpes family. Its highest incidence is between the years of 15 and 25. Infectious mononucleosis (mono) is more common among college students than the general population, especially in early spring and fall.

One attack of infectious mononucleosis is believed to offer permanent immunity but there are a few rare exceptions. There are many people with documented mononucleosis who give a past history of the disease; however, the previous diagnosis frequently was based on the clinical findings and did not include laboratory data. Assessment of infectious mononucleosis should be based on three criteria: clinical findings (pharyngitis and posterior cervical lymphadenopathy), blood work (atypical lymphocytes, positive heterophil antibody titer, and elevated liver function tests), and a positive screening test for EBv.

The disease is spread by intimate contact with an infected person. Contrary to public opinion, this is not a very contagious disease even among family members. The virus is found in the nasopharyngeal tract from one week to several months after the illness.

The clinical course of mono may vary from a very mild to a severe illness. The average duration of illness is between two to four weeks. It is believed that many cases are so mild, especially in young children, that the assessment of infectious mononucleosis is never made. This may explain why transmission of the disease is so difficult.

HISTORY

The onset is generally abrupt. The patient first notices malaise and fatigue. Frequently, a student will complain of difficulty concentrating on course work. The malaise and fatigue is followed by complaints of a sore throat, irregular fever (100° to 101°F), and swollen glands, especially in the neck. The fever is present for one to two weeks.

PHYSICAL EXAMINATION

More than 90% of people with infectious mononucleosis have pharyngitis and cervical lymphadenopathy. If the tonsils are present, they often have a dirty white exudate. Since the anterior cervical chain is associated in the majority of sore throats, it is the posterior cervical chain involvement that is the important physical finding.

Abdominal organ enlargement is not an uncommon clinical finding. Approximately 50% of clients have an enlarged spleen that can be palpated on the seventh day of the illness. Since the spleen's capsule is weakened, aggressive palpation and strenuous physical activity should be avoided. The greatest risk of splenic rupture is between the tenth and twenty-first days. About 15% have liver enlargement and less than 5% have clinical jaundice.

Occasionally, there is a pale, transient, red maculopapular rash. The rash is similar to a rubella rash except it tends to spare the face. The rash is present early in the clinical course and in less than 5% of the cases.

DIAGNOSTIC TESTS

Since the clinical findings of mononucleosis are similar to many other infectious diseases, an accurate assessment must be based on laboratory as well as clinical data. The following are the laboratory tests used in making the assessment of infectious mononucleosis.

White Blood Count (WBC). The WBC is elevated to between 10,000 to 20,000 per cubic millimeter with greater than 50% lymphocytes. Many of the lymphocytes have an atypical form (Downey cells) which are not pathognomonic since they are also present in other viral illnesses.

Heterophil Antibody Titer. During the second week of the illness, this titer begins to rise. After six weeks, there is a gradual fall.

Liver Function Tests. The results of the liver function tests are mildly elevated. These tests include alkaline phosphatase, serum glutamic-oxaloacetic transaminase (SGOT), and serum glutamic-pyruvic transaminase (SGPT).

Mono Spot Test. This test has positive results as the number of antibodies to the EBv increase. A positive test is usually not present until the second week of the illness and may continue to be positive up to six months.

Throat Culture. Throat culture is recommended to rule out Beta-hemolytic streptococci.

MANAGEMENT

Since infectious mononucleosis is a viral illness, there is no specific treatment. Its management needs to include client education and supportive and symptomatic care.

Counseling

Client education is the key to the management of infectious mononucleosis. For an uneventful, rapid recovery, in addition to supportive and symptomatic measures, the client and often the parents need to have a good understanding of the disease process. Educating clients on the following information is essential:

1. Only intimate contacts are at real risk of becoming ill, not dormitory roommates.

2. Bed rest is recommended for three to five days. Students can usually return to their classes after one week. After three to four weeks, most clients can return to full activity. The exception is athletes; since the danger of splenic rupture exists, athletics should be avoided for four weeks.

3. Symptoms last about two weeks; however, fatigue may continue for three to four months. Adequate rest (at least eight hours of sleep) and good nutrition are important.

4. Until the liver function tests return to normal, alcohol should be avoided. If the patient had clinical jaundice, alcohol should be avoided for 6 to 12 months.

5. Stress that infectious mononucleosis is a viral disease and antibiotics are ineffective against viruses.

Pharmacology

Medications play a minor role in management of infectious mononucleosis. Analgesics and antipyretics are given for fever and myalgia. If the throat culture is positive of group A beta-hemolytic *Streptococcus,* antibiotics are necessary. (See Acute Pharyngitis).

Referral

Consultation and/or referral is recommended for clients with clinical jaundice or whose illness continues beyond two months.

ACUTE SINUSITIS

Since the mucous membranes of the nose are continuous with those of the accessory nasal sinuses (frontal, maxillary, sphenoid, and ethmoid), any infection of the nose usually will involve one or more of these sinuses. However, this is not acute sinusitis. Acute sinusitis is diagnosed when infection in one of the paranasal sinuses is the major clinical finding.

Acute sinusitis results from inadequate drainage of sinus secretions. This may be secondary to an obstructive process (polyps, deviated septum, hypertrophic turbinates), abrupt intranasal pressure changes (diving, deep swimming), chronic rhinitis, maxillary dental abscess, or acute infections of the nose.

At birth, only two sinuses are large enough to harbor infections: the maxil-

Table 5.1. Sinus Involvement, Location of Pain and Complications

Sinus	Pain Location	Complications
Frontal	Forehead, above eyebrows	Brain abscess Osteomyelitis Subdural empyema
Maxillary	Upper teeth and cheeks	Osteomyelitis (rare)
Ethmoid	Temples, over eyes Distribution of trigeminal nerve	Meningitis, cavernous sinus thrombosis
Sphenoid	Suboccipital	Meningitis, cavernous sinus thrombosis

lary and the ethmoid. The sphenoidal and frontal sinuses do not develop enough to cause clinical problems until about age 4 and 7, respectively. The organisms most frequently responsible for acute sinusitis are *Hemophilus influenzae, Pneumococcus, Staphylococcus, Streptococcus,* and the coryzavirus.

Sinusitis is not as common in children as it is in adults. However, the complications are just as serious. Complications arise when the infected sinus is unable to drain into the nasal chamber and the infection burrows out of the sinus cavity (see Table 5.1).

HISTORY

The onset of sinusitis can be gradual or sudden. Frequently, it occurs three to five days after a viral upper respiratory infection. The dominant complaint is headache. The sinus headache is described as worse in the morning and disappearing by midafternoon. The facial pain is usually localized to the anatomical position of the involved sinus (see Table 5.1). Other symptoms reported are tearing, nasal obstruction, increased nasal discharge, periorbital edema, fever, and malaise.

PHYSICAL

Inspection of the nose reveals an erythematous, swollen mucosa with a profuse mucopurulent discharge. However, if obstruction is complete, there may be no discharge. Tenderness usually is present over the sinus involved. If the maxillary or frontal sinus is involved, transillumination may assist in the location of the infection. Oral temperatures are usually less than 103°F.

DIAGNOSTIC TESTS

A reliable assessment can be based on a careful clinical history and physical examination. However, in those cases where the signs and symptoms are less well-defined, white blood cell count (WBC), nasal smears, and roentgenograms of the sinuses may be helpful. Expected results are as follows:

1. WBC may be normal or mildly elevated.
2. Nasal smear. Allergy is suspected when large numbers of eosinophils are found. An infectious cause is associated with polymorphonuclear leukocytes.
3. Roentgenograms of the sinuses may show hazy cloudiness and/or fluid level in the affected sinus.

MANAGEMENT

The three goals in the management of acute sinus infection are to establish drainage, combat the bacterial infection, and relieve the pain.

Counseling

Establishing good drainage is the key to a rapid recovery. The following supportive therapy is recommended for educating parents who have children with sinusitis:

1. Use hot wet towels to midface and forehead for one to two hours, four times a day.
2. Encourage adequate hydration by having children double their usual fluid intake.
3. If nasal secretions are thick, nasal irrigation with normal saline will help promote drainage.
4. Place a vaporizer close enough to the child so that bed clothes become damp. This will keep inspired air moist and respiratory secretions thinner.

Pharmacology

Medications are used in the management of acute sinusitis to restore the ostia, relieve pain and fever, and combat infection. Antibiotics alone will not suffice. Unless the infected sinus can drain, the infection will not heal.

1. Analgesics and antipyretics. Aspirin and/or acetaminophen are given for fever and myalgia.
2. Topical nasal decongestants. Use of topical nasal decongestants (e.g. Afrin Nasal Spray) is controversial due to ciliary stasis and rebound hyperemia.
3. Systemic decongestants. Oral decongestants with or without antihistamines are used to promote drainage. However, antihistamines should be used cautiously as they can result in too much drying of secretions and actually inhibit drainage.
4. Antibiotics. Penicillin, erythromycin, and ampicillin are the drugs of choice.

Referral

As previously stated, complications arise when the infected sinus is unable to drain and the infection extends past the sinus. Complications of sinusitis, although rare, are associated with high morbidity and mortality. Increased headaches, nausea and vomiting, distortion of vision, signs of increasing intracranial pressure, leucocytosis (WBC> 20,000 per cu mm), and systemic toxicity are danger signs for serious complications. An immediate referral is indicated if complications are suspected.

INFLUENZA

Influenza is a major public health problem. During an epidemic, as high as 50% of the general public have been affected. The morbidity and mortality associated with influenza can be very high in certain at-risk children.

There are three types of influenzae (Types A, B, and C). Type A is responsible for the more severe and widespread epidemic outbreaks of the disease. On the other hand, Type B produces a milder illness and only localized spread. Type B is sometimes incorrectly referred to as the common cold. Type C is rarely responsible for disease. This chapter will only discuss Type A influenza.

One of the major difficulties with Type A influenza is its ability to alter its surface proteins. This means that the virus is capable of mutating itself to produce a new strain. Therefore, antibodies that were acquired (naturally or vaccine-induced) to the old virus are now rendered either weak or noneffective against this new strain.

The virus is shed from the nasopharyngeal tract, therefore, spread by direct contact with an affected person. The child is ill for approximately three days but is contagious up to four days after the onset of symptoms. Since the incubation period is only two days, it is no wonder that Type A influenza spreads so rapidly.

HISTORY AND PHYSICAL EXAMINATION

Sudden onset of fever, sore throat, cough, headache, general malaise and loss of appetite are not uncommon. However, the onset may be gradual. Oral temperatures range from low-grade to as high as 106°F.

Certain children are considered high risk, and are more prone to develop complications, particularly pneumococcal pneumonia. High-risk children include those who are immunosuppressed and have a chronic disease (metabolic disorders or pulmonary or cardiac disease). Other rare complications of influenza are Reye's syndrome, meningitis, myocarditis, hemorrhagic epistaxis, and hematemesis.

MANAGEMENT

If a healthy child contracts influenza, only supportive and symptomatic treatment is useful. As with all viral illnesses, antibiotics are not effective unless signs of a secondary bacterial superinfection are present. Therefore, the nurse practitioner should advise antipyretics (acetaminophen is preferred; aspirin has been linked to causing Reye's syndrome with influenza) to control fever, encourage adequate fluid intake to prevent dehydration, and advise rest.

In the high-risk population, prevention of influenza through vaccine programs is the goal. However, there are many myths regarding the influenza vaccine; a few are based on facts while the majority are not. It is the nurse practitioner's responsibility to provide education regarding the advantages and limitations of the influenza vaccine.

Referral

Consultation with a physician is advised for high-risk children who contract Type A influenza. Referral is indicated for children who develop complications.

STUDY QUESTIONS

Circle all that apply.

1. Which of the following physical findings would be indicative of an acute otitis media?

a. erythema involving more than 30% of the tympanic membrane
b. an immobile, retracted tympanic membrane with circumferential erythema
c. flaky white debris on the surface of the tympanic membrane
d. an immobile, bulging tympanic membrane

2. Symptoms of acute otitis media in the 1-year-old child may include which of the following?

a. diarrhea
b. anorexia
c. temperature of 39°C
d. vomiting
e. all of above

A 3-year-old boy is awakened from sleep with pain in the right ear. His mother notes a rectal temperature of 37° C (98.6° F) and decides to treat the youngster with acetaminophen and analgesic ear drops. The next morning the child is no better and has a temperature of 39° C (102.4° F).

3. The most common causative organisms of otitis media at this age are:

a. *H. influenzae* and *D. pneumoniae*
b. *Streptococcus* and *Staphylococcus*
c. *E. coli* and *D. pneumoniae*
d. *Staphylococcus* and *H. influenzae*

Ann has an essentially normal physical examination except for boggy nasal mucosa, purulent nasal discharge and purulent postnasal drainage. Ann's mother asks you to give her a penicillin shot to "cure" her cold.

4. Which of the following statements might be given as an answer to Ann's mother?

a. antibiotics kill or arrest the growth of bacteria, but have no effect on viruses
b. harmful and nonharmful bacteria coexist within the body. The nonharmful bacteria keep harmful organisms under control, but since antibiotics kill the bacteria indiscriminately, they permit harmful bacteria to overgrow and cause illness
c. antibiotics given indiscriminately encourage the development of resistant strains of bacteria
d. antibiotics may result in allergic or toxic reactions which can prove harmful

5. Six-year-old Bobby has complained of a sore throat for 24 hours. Yesterday, when he came home from school, he complained of a headache and
   abdominal pain. He vomited after supper and had a temperature of 101°F
   orally. By morning, he refused to eat, saying that he could not swallow.
   The management of Bobby's complaints should include:

   a. counseling
   b. throat culture
   c. aspirin every two to three hours
   d. warm saline gargles

6. Major complications of streptococcal infections are:

   a. rheumatic fever
   b. rheumatoid arthritis
   c. acute glomerulonephritis
   d. hemolytic anemia

7. Which of the following complications is *unlikely* to occur in influenza A
   infections?

   a. bacterial pneumonia
   b. jaundice
   c. myocarditis
   d. meningitis
   e. respiratory failure due to primary influenza virus pneumonia

8. A 19-year-old college student has a severe sore throat, a temperature of
   102° F, and has had general malaise for two weeks. His tonsils are moderately red with gray-white exudate. Cervical lymphadenopathy is evident in the posterior cervical chain. A diffuse maculopapular rash is
   noted. What is the probable infecting organism?

   a. Epstein-Barr virus
   b. gonococcus
   c. *Streptococcus pyogenes*
   d. adenovirus

9. Complications of an acute sinusitis are rare. Which of the following is
   not a danger signal for acute sinusitis?

   a. increased headache pain
   b. facial pain
   c. distortion of vision
   d. nausea and vomiting

10. Thirteen-year-old Mary is on the swim team at school. Yesterday morning she began to have a dull pain in her left ear. This morning the pain is less severe and the left ear is draining. The best assessment is a:

    a. left maxillary sinusitis
    b. left external otitis
    c. left perforated tympanic membrane
    d. left mastoiditis

ANSWERS

1. d	6. a, c
2. e	7. b
3. a	8. a
4. a, b, c, d	9. b
5. a, b, d	10. c

BIBLIOGRAPHY

Cummings, C. W., & Treyve, E. L. Common mouth and throat infections. *Hospital Medicine*, January, 87.

Fletcher, M. M. The painful ear. *Medical Times*, September 1978, *106*, 29.

Giebink, G. S., Mills, E. L., & Huff, J. S. The microbiology of serous and mucoid otitis media. *Pediatrics*, 1979, *63*, 915.

Holliday, M. J., & Michael, J. Some common ear problems. *Hospital Medicine*, May 1981, 13.

Kilbourne, E. D., & Edwin, D. Influenza pandemics in perspective. *JAMA*, 1977, *237*, 1225.

Leveque, H., & Fletcher, M. M. I have sinus trouble! *Medical Times*, September 1978, *106*, 9.

Middleton, D. B. A logical approach to managing sore throats. *Modern Medicine*, November 30, 1980, 40.

Morgan, P. R. Sinusitis: a headache with fatal possibilities. *Modern Medicine*, September 1981.

Nolen, J. W. Infectious mononucleosis. *The Nurse Practitioner Journal*, March-April 1979, 2.

Pons, V. G., & Dolin, R. Influenza. *Hospital Medicine,* October 1978, 15.

Shields, C. E. Infectious mononucleosis as a student health problem. *JCAM,* October 1979.

Shurin, P. A., Pelton, S. I., & Donner, A. Persistence of middle ear effusion after acute otitis media in children. *New England Journal of Medicine,* 1979, *300,* 1121.

CHAPTER 6

MIDDLE AND LOWER RESPIRATORY INFECTIONS

Beverly Bitterman

Pediatric middle and lower respiratory tract infections can be viral or bacterial in nature. Those commonly seen by the nurse practitioner in an ambulatory setting include laryngotracheobronchitis, epiglottitis, bronchitis, bronchiolitis, and pneumonia.

LARYNGOTRACHEOBRONCHITIS

Laryngotracheobronchitis, commonly known as croup, is a viral infection that causes inflammation and edema of the larynx, trachea, and bronchi. This edema is responsible for the characteristic inspiratory stridor, hoarseness, and cough. Two-thirds of all cases of croup are caused by the parainfluenza virus and occur in late fall and early winter. The remaining one-third of cases are caused by the adenovirus, respiratory syncytial virus, influenza virus, and rubeola virus. Viral croup occurs in children between the ages of 3 months and 5 years, with the majority of cases occurring under 3 years.

HISTORY AND PHYSICAL EXAMINATION

On physical exam, the child usually does not appear seriously ill. There is a barky, "croupy" cough and history of an upper respiratory infection (URI) with conjunctivitis and/or rhinorrhea. As the infection progresses, inspiratory stridor, with increasing respiratory difficulty and retractions, develops.

The expiratory phase of respiration becomes prolonged. The child will have diminished breath sounds at the lung bases with scattered rales, rhonchi, and wheezing. The temperature will usually be 38 to 39° C. Symptoms are reported to be worse at night. Frequently, there is a family history of a recent respiratory illness.

Acute spasmodic laryngitis, a variant of acute laryngotracheobronchitis, occurs most commonly in children between the ages of 1 and 3 years. The cause is usually viral; however, it may be allergic or psychologic. The onset of spasmodic croup is sudden and occurs most frequently in the evening or nighttime. There may be a client/family history of a recent upper respiratory infection. The child awakens with a barky cough and inspiratory stridor. Symptoms frequently decrease on the way to the emergency room as the child is exposed to the cool night air.

A detailed history is indicated to distinguish between the forms of viral croup and other possible causes of upper airway obstruction. Physician consultation is needed if the diagnosis is unclear. The primary concern is assessment of the degree of respiratory distress. The differential diagnosis includes epiglottitis, aspiration of a foreign body, retropharyngeal abscess, external compression of the airway, intraluminal obstruction from masses, angioneurotic edema, postendotracheal intubation, hypocalcemic tetany, infectious mononucleosis, trauma, and asthma.

DIAGNOSTIC TESTS

Although most assessments are made by the clinical history and physical exam alone, occasionally it is necessary to utilize laboratory values and roentgenograms when a clear diagnosis of laryngotracheobronchitis or spasmodic laryngitis cannot be made. Expected results of the more commonly utilized diagnostic tests are as follows:

1. WBC> 15,000/cu mm with no significant shift to the left
2. Negative blood cultures
3. X-ray film of the cervical trachea shows fixed circumferential subglottic narrowing
4. Chest roentgenogram is normal

MANAGEMENT

Outpatient management is possible for children without inspiratory stridor at rest. Children with symptoms of increasing airway obstruction need to be referred for hospitalization. Symptoms of impending obstruction include tachypnea (rate > 60/minute), cyanosis, restlessness, and increased intercostal retractions. Late signs of respiratory failure include listlessness and a decrease in stridor and retractions without clinical improvement. This requires immediate respiratory assistance.

Counseling

Outpatient management of the child with croup includes the following supportive measures:

1. Educate the caretaker on symptoms of increasing respiratory obstruction.
2. Place a cool mist vaporizer close enough to the child so that the night clothes become damp.
3. Place the child in a steamy bathroom for 15 to 20 minute intervals several times a day.
4. Encourage oral fluids (room temperature clear liquids) to promote optimum hydration as determined by good skin turgor and adequate amounts of light yellow urine.
5. Maintain a calm atmosphere to prevent increased oxygen requirements due to crying.
6. Elevate the child's upper body by an infant seat or pillows.

Pharmacology

Antipyretics (acetaminophen or aspirin) are used to control temperatures of 102°F or greater and promote comfort. Since aspirin has been linked to Reye's Syndrome, acetaminophen has become the drug of choice in viral illnesses. If necessary to control the fever, aspirin and acetaminophen may be alternated so that the child is receiving an antipyretic every two hours.

1. Acetaminophen (Tempra, Tylenol): Infants, 10 mg/kg/dose in 6 doses (every 3–4 hours); 1–3 years, 60–120 mg/kg/dose; 6–12 years, 240 mg/kg/dose; 12 years and older, 300–600 mg/kg/dose.
2. Aspirin: 65 mg/year of age/dose in 6 doses (every 4 hours); 10 years and older, 300–600 mg/kg/dose

REFERRAL

Hospitalization is indicated in conditions with threatening airway obstruction, low blood oxygen levels, and inability to maintain adequate oral intake. The nurse practitioner will need to refer the client if hospitalization should become indicated.

Prognosis of children with tracheolaryngeobronchitis is good, as most children do not develop airway obstruction and recover within three to seven days. If death occurs, it is generally secondary to laryngeal obstruction or from complications of a tracheotomy.

EPIGLOTTITIS

Epiglottitis is a bacterial infection of the epiglottis, aryepiglottic folds, and supraglottic area that causes airway obstruction. Epiglottitis is a pediatric emergency affecting children between the ages of 3 and 7 years. It is most frequently caused by *Hemophilus influenza* type B and is often accompanied by septicemia. There does not seem to be a seasonal incidence of this disease.

HISTORY AND PHYSICAL EXAMINATION

The onset of epiglottitis is sudden, with only 25% of children experiencing a preceding minor respiratory illness. Older children may complain of a sore throat and dysphagia that rapidly progresses to respiratory distress. Generally, there is no family history of respiratory illness.

    The child appears pale, toxic, and lethargic. The voice may be muffled but not hoarse. Drooling is common. Fever may be 39.4° C. (103° F.), or higher. A cough is rare. Breathing difficulty increases in two to four hours with signs of obstruction being the same as for viral croup; for example tachypnea, stridor at rest, retractions, restlessness leading to listlessness, cyanosis, and respiratory failure. Direct visualization of the epiglottis should be attempted only when intubation is intended, since it is possible to stimulate sudden, complete obstruction. This procedure is generally performed by a physician trained in intubation. The epiglottis will appear edematous and cherry red.

DIAGNOSTIC TESTS

Laboratory values and roentgenograms can help establish a firm diagnosis and rule out other causes of respiratory obstruction, such as croup, foreign body aspiration, and trauma. The expected results of commonly ordered diagnostic tests are as follows:

1. WBC > 18,000/cu mm with a shift to the left
2. Blood cultures positive for *H. influenzae* type B

3. Soft tissue roentgenograms of the lateral neck may confirm the enlargement of the epiglottis
4. Chest roentgenogram is normal

MANAGEMENT

A child with epiglottitis needs to be stabilized and transported to an acute care medical facility. Intubation must be done in a setting where someone capable of performing a tracheotomy is available, if obstruction should become complete. Before or during transport, the nurse practitioner should establish an intravenous line, draw a blood culture, and begin parenteral ampicillin (300 mg/kg/day in six divided doses). The child should be kept in an upright position for transport. If attendants are not able to intubate, a large bore needle should be carried in the event that obstruction becomes complete and an emergency cricoidotomy is needed.

Mortality may be as high as 50% without intubation. With proper management, however, prognosis is good. The child is usually extubated within two to three days.

BRONCHITIS

Bronchitis, an inflammation of the bronchi, is of viral origin and occurs most commonly with an upper respiratory tract infection. It also may be associated with influenza, pertussis, measles, and scarlet fever. In older children and adolescents, an acute, primary, undifferentiated viral tracheobronchitis can occur.

HISTORY AND PHYSICAL EXAMINATION

Frequently, there is a history of an upper respiratory infection. The child may have a dry, racking, nonproductive cough which began three to four days after the onset of rhinitis. A burning chest pain aggravated by coughing is commonly reported. This may be followed by noisy breath sounds and, occasionally, shortness of breath. General malaise is accompanied by a low-grade fever. The cough may become productive and change from clear to purulent. In five to ten days the mucus thins and the cough begins to decrease. Physical findings vary with the age of the child and the stage of the disease. Breath sounds may be clear or coarse with presence of rales and high pitched rhonchi.

DIAGNOSTIC TESTS

Laboratory and radiologic tests are not usually necessary to establish the diagnosis of bronchitis. If the diagnosis is unclear, physician consultation is indicated. Differential diagnoses include asthma, respiratory tract anomaly, foreign body, obstruction, bronchiectasis, immune deficiency, tuberculosis, allergy, sinusitis, tonsillitis, adenoiditis, pneumonia, and cystic fibrosis. Results of the most commonly used diagnostic tests are as follows:

1. WBC is normal or slightly elevated
2. Chest roentgenogram may be normal or show increased bronchovesicular markings

MANAGEMENT

As bronchitis is generally viral, treatment is supportive and symptomatic. Parent education is the key to a rapid recovery.

Counseling

The goal of bronchitis management is to promote hydration and drainage. Stressing to the parents that it is usually a viral illness and does not generally require an antibiotic is essential. Also, it is important to educate parents on the following supportive therapy:

1. Use of postural drainage to facilitate pulmonary drainage
2. Encourage increased oral fluids (room temperature clear liquids) to promote optimum hydration as determined by good skin turgor and adequate amounts of light yellow urine
3. Place a cool mist vaporizer close enough to the child so that the bedclothes become damp. This will keep inspired air moist and help sooth the irritated throat and respiratory tract.
4. The child may be more comfortable propped at a 30° to 40° angle. Infants may be placed in an infant seat.

Pharmacology

Since bronchitis is generally a viral illness, medications play a minor role in its management. As stated previously, the goal of bronchitis therapy is to promote hydration and drainage. Since antihistamines dry secretions, they should not be used. Cough suppressants should be used only if the cough is interfering with the child's sleep. An effective antitussive may be made from equal parts of lemon juice, honey, and whiskey (give 1 to 2 teaspoons at bedtime).

Antibiotics should be used only if bacterial complications are suspected, or if the child's cough has continued into the third week. Signs of bacterial complications include onset of a sudden, high fever, worsening cough, purulent productive sputum, and a high WBC. Erythromycin (50 mg/kg/24 hours) is the antibiotic of choice.

If the fever is high and/or causing discomfort, antipyretics may be used. Acetaminophen (Tempra, Tylenol) and aspirin are commonly used and may be alternated so that the child receives one of the antipyretics every two hours. Acetaminophen is given as follows: infants, 10 mg/kg/dose every four to six hours; 1–3 years, 60–120 mg/kg/dose; 3–6 years, 120 mg/kg/dose; 6–12 years, 240 mg/kg/dose; 12 years and older, 300–600 mg/kg/dose. Aspirin is given as follows: 65 mg/year of age/dose up to 650 mg every four to six hours.

Referral

Children who do not respond to the above therapy, or have repeated attacks of acute bronchitis need to be referred to a physician.

BRONCHIOLITIS

Acute bronchiolitis is a disease resulting from bronchiolar obstruction due to edema and mucus accumulation. It is caused primarily by the respiratory syncytial virus. Other causative agents are the parainfluenza 3 virus, mycoplasma, and some adenoviruses. Bronchiolar obstruction leads to increased airway resistance, air trapping, and overinflation. Atelectasis may occur. Diminished ventilation of the alveoli may result in hypoxemia. Carbon dioxide retention is an increased risk as respirations exceed 60 per minute. Bronchiolitis is more common during the winter months and in children 2 years of age.

HISTORY AND PHYSICAL EXAMINATION

History of recent exposure to older children or adults with mild respiratory diseases is common. The infant initially has a mild upper respiratory infection with rhinorrhea, a fever of 38.5° to 39° C. (101° to 102° F.), and decreased appetite. These symptoms may last from one to three days. A gradual development of respiratory distress with a paroxysmal wheezy cough, dyspnea, and increased irritability follow. Both bottle and breastfeeding may be difficult due to tachypnea. Air hunger and cyanosis may be present along with intercostal and subcostal retractions. The liver and spleen may be palpable below the costal margins as the diaphragm becomes depressed due to emphysema. Auscultation reveals wheezing; scattered fine rales may be heard at the end of inspiration and at the beginning of expiration. The expiratory phase of respiration becomes prolonged.

Bronchiolitis may be confused with bronchial asthma. The following factors favor the diagnosis of asthma: a positive family history for asthma, eosinophilia, repeated attacks, sudden onset without a preceding infection, and a favorable response to a dose of epinephrine (0.01 ml/kg of 1:1000 dilution given subcutaneously). Other differential diagnoses include congestive heart failure, foreign body in the trachea, pertussis, bacterial bronchopneumonias, and cystic fibrosis.

DIAGNOSTIC TESTS

In addition to the history and physical examination, the following diagnostic tests may be helpful in establishing the diagnosis of bronchiolitis:

1. WBC and differential are generally within normal limits.
2. Chest roentgenogram may be clear except for hyperexpansion with an increased anteroposterior diameter on lateral view. One-third of the infants will have scattered areas of consolidation.

MANAGEMENT

Supportive therapy as outlined under the section on bronchitis, is instituted. Hospitalization is indicated for infants with respiratory distress.

The infant is generally most ill during the first two to three days after the onset of cough and dyspnea. After the third day, recovery is rapid with less than a 1% mortality rate. Death may occur due to dehydration, apnea, or severe uncompensated respiratory acidosis.

PNEUMONIA

Pneumonia is acute inflammation of the lung alveoli. The disease may be caused by several different pathogens. Approximately 50% of childhood pneumonias are caused by viral agents and occur during seasonal epidemics.

The most common viral agents are respiratory syncytial virus, parainfluenza viruses, adenovirus, and enterovirus. *Mycoplasma pneumoniae* is thought to be responsible for 40 to 60% of pneumonia cases among school-aged children. Other frequent causative agents include *Chlamydia* and *Pneumococcus*. It is necessary to use diagnostic tests to establish the differential diagnosis. Besides the type of pneumonia, bronchiolitis, asthma, cystic fibrosis, and other causes of pulmonary infiltrates, (e.g., mycobacteria, fungi, and neoplasms) should be considered.

VIRAL PNEUMONIAS

History and Physical Examination

Children with viral pneumonias generally have a history of upper respiratory infection with several days of cough and rhinitis. There also may be a history of an upper respiratory infection in other family members. The child's symptoms progress slowly until he/she develops tachypnea, a cough that may be dry or productive, with blood-tinged or purulent sputum, retractions, decreased breath sounds, rales, and wheezing. The child may appear cyanotic. The severity of the illness depends somewhat on the age of the child, general health, and the viral agent. Viral pneumonias can be very severe in young infants. The older child will not appear as acutely ill as his fever indicates. The temperature may be as high as 40° C. (104° F.), however, the pulse is generally not above 100 per minute.

Diagnostic Tests

The following are the results of several commonly ordered tests as they would appear in the diagnosis of viral pneumonia:

1. The WBC is generally normal or slightly elevated, but not higher than 20,000/cu mm.
2. Platelets may be slightly depressed.
3. Chest roentgenogram characteristically shows diffuse patchy densities, especially in the perihilar areas. Effusion may occur.

Management

The nurse practitioner should consult with the physician preceptor in the treatment of any child with pneumonia. The principles of the management of viral pneumonia are the same as for bronchitis. They include promotion of rest, hydration, adequate nutrition, antipyretics for temperature control, maintenance of patent airway, and monitoring of respiratory status and vital signs for indications of complications. Infants under 6 months of age and other infants and children with severe viral pneumonias need to be hospitalized for closer supervision.

MYCOPLASMA PNEUMONIAS

Mycoplasmas are bacteria that lack a cell wall. The greatest incidence of *Mycoplasma* pneumonias is between 5 and 19 years. It is often difficult to differentiate between viral and *Mycoplasma* pneumonias. *Mycoplasma* pneumonias occur throughout the year with increased incidence in the summer and fall months. This is in contrast to viral pneumonias which tend to occur with viral epidemics during the winter months; viral pneumonias are often preceded by an upper respiratory infection. *Mycoplasma* pneumonias are mildly contagious, infecting about 30% of susceptible family members.

History and Physical Examination

A severe frontal headache suggests *Mycoplasma* rather than viral pneumonia. Other presenting symptoms include a cough which increases in severity, small amounts of blood-flecked sputum, low grade fever of 38.5° C. (101° F.), malaise, sore throat, and poor appetite. The child is often brought to the nurse practitioner because a seemingly common cold has failed to resolve. Scattered rales are often auscultated over bilateral lung fields. Pharyngitis, otitis media, and bullous myringitis may be found. There will be a rash in 10 to 20% of the cases, generally involving the upper body, arms, and legs. It may also involve oral and conjunctival mucosa. The rash is noncharacteristic and can appear in nearly all forms.

Diagnostic Tests

The following are the findings from helpful diagnostic tests:

1. WBC is normal or mildly elevated.
2. Cold agglutinin titer is 1:32 or greater in 50% of the cases. The titer may be negative in early disease and positive after 7 to 10 days of infection.
3. Chest roentgenogram findings are variable and often more impressive than clinical findings from the chest examination. They may show diffuse patchy densities, especially in the perihilar areas or segmental lower lobe consolidation with pleural fluids.

Management

Although *Mycoplasma* rarely proceeds to dangerous pneumonia, antibiotic therapy is indicated since it shortens the course of the disease. Tetracycline is the drug of choice. Erythromycin is also effective and is the drug of choice in small children because tetracycline discolors developing teeth. Erythromycin also has the advantage of being effective against pneumococcal pneumonia. Tetracycline (25–50 mg/kg/24 hours in four doses up to the adult dose of 250–500 mg/dose) or erythromycin (50 mg/kg/24 hours in six doses up to the adult dose of 250 mg/dose) is given for 7 to 10 days. Symptomatic treatment, as outlined under the section on bronchitis, is instituted. Hospitalization usually is not necessary.

BACTERIAL PNEUMONIA

Pneumococcal pneumonia is responsible for over 90% of childhood bacterial pneumonias. Other pathogens include *Streptococcus, Staphylococcus,* and *H. influenzae.* These infections occur most frequently, although not exclusively, in late winter and early spring in children under 5 years of age. Bacterial pneumonias occur more frequently in children with another underlying disease, an upper respiratory infection, or a childhood exanthem.

History and Physical Examination

The onset of the pneumonia is rapid. The child becomes febrile with a temperature of 39.4° to 40° C. (103° to 104° F.). Tachycardia to a rate of 140 to 160 and tachypnea to a rate of 50 to 80 respirations per minute commonly develop. Older children complain of a headache and chills. Infants may have vomiting or diarrhea and may have convulsions at the onset. A dry cough and dyspnea are present. Dullness may be noted on percussion. Chest auscultation may be normal or reveal diminished breath sounds and fine crackling.

Diagnostic Tests

The expected results of commonly utilized diagnostic tests are as follows:

1. WBC is elevated above 10,000/cu mm and may be as high as 40,000/cu mm with a shift to the left
2. Chest roentgenogram shows dense segmental or lobar infiltrate that is usually unilateral
3. Blood culture may also reveal the organism

Management

Bacterial pneumonia should be primarily managed by a physician. Most young infants must be hospitalized. Older infants and children may be managed at home, depending on the severity of the illness and the home situation. Supportive care (see section on bronchitis) is instituted. Antibiotic therapy is indicated and is specific for the cultured organism and its sensitivity. Penicillin is the treatment of choice for pneumococcal pneumonia. A single injection of procaine penicillin (300,000 to 600,000 units) is followed by oral penicillin (50,000 units/kg/24 hours) for 10 days.

STUDY QUESTIONS

Circle all that apply.

1. Mrs. Lock calls you at 9 PM and tells you that her 3-year-old son, Johnny, is having trouble breathing. Which of the following history questions would you ask? (Choose all that apply.)

   a. When did the difficulty start?
   b. Has he had a cold?
   c. How fast is he breathing?
   d. Does he seem to be getting air in?
   e. Are any family members sick?
   f. What is his temperature?
   g. Is he drooling?
   h. Does he have a cough?

2. You are thinking about several possible diagnoses. It is most important to rule out the following possibility first:

   a. acute epiglottitis
   b. laryngotracheobronchitis
   c. spasmodic laryngitis
   d. viral pneumonia

3. You find out that Johnny woke up from a sound sleep with a harsh cough. He had not been sick. No family members are ill. He is getting air in but it is taking "all his strength." He is not drooling. His temperature is 101° F. (rectal). Your best assessment from this information is:

   a. acute epiglottitis
   b. laryngotracheobronchitis

    c. spasmodic laryngitis

    d. aspiration of foreign body

4. After physical examination and diagnostic tests have been completed you establish that Johnny has spasmodic laryngitis. List several supportive measures used with any respiratory illness.

    a.

    b.

    c.

    d.

    e.

5. Antibiotic therapy is indicated for which four of the following pediatric illnesses?

    a. acute epiglottitis

    b. laryngotracheobronchitis

    c. spasmodic laryngitis

    d. acute bronchitis

    e. acute bronchiolitis

    f. viral pneumonia

    g. mycoplasma pneumonia

    h. chlamydial pneumonia

    i. pneumococcal pneumonia

6. Two-year-old Tammy is brought to the clinic by her grandmother. She has a two-day history of poor appetite, wheezing cough, difficulty breathing, and fever of 100.8° F. (rectal). On physical examination you note that she appears to be in moderate respiratory distress with retractions and circumoral cyanosis. Auscultation reveals wheezing over all lobes. The two most probable diagnoses are:

    a. viral pneumonia

    b. bronchitis

    c. bronchiolitis

    d. bronchial asthma

7. A good way to establish the correct diagnosis with Tammy is to:

    a. order a chest x-ray film

    b. give epinephrine (0.01 ml/kg of 1:1000 dilution subcutaneously)

    c. order a WBC

8. Which of the following pneumonias are most likely to be preceded by an upper respiratory infection?

   a. viral
   b. pneumococcal
   c. mycoplasmal
   d. chlamydial

9. Chlamydial pneumonia is most common in which age group?

   a. 3 to 12 weeks
   b. 1 to 3 years
   c. 3 to 6 years
   d. 5 to 20 years

10. You are given the results from diagnostic tests done on 3-year-old you have never seen. They are:

   a. WBC, 30,000 with a shift to the left
   b. chest roentgenogram, left lower lobe infiltrate

Based on these tests, your best guess of the diagnosis is:

   a. viral pneumonia
   b. mycoplasmal pneumonia
   c. chlamydial pneumonia
   d. bacterial pneumonia

11. Your examination reveals a very sick child with a temperature of 103° F. (rectal), respiratory rate of 50/minute, and heart rate of 150/minute. Chest auscultation reveals diminished breath sounds. Select one of the following managements:

   a. begin penicillin V (50,000 units/kg/24 hours)
   b. begin erythromycin (50 mg/kg/24 hours)
   c. perform cricoidotomy
   d. refer

ANSWERS

1. all air
2. a
3. c
4. a. education regarding signs of increasing respiratory distress

   b. humidification of inspired air
   c. increased oral fluids
   d. calm, soothing atmosphere
   e. antipyretics for fever and malaise
   f. elevation of the child's upper body

5. a, g, h, and i

6. c and d

7. b

8. a and b

9. a

10. d

11. d

BIBLIOGRAPHY

Barker, G. A. Current management of croup and epiglottitis. *The Pediatric Clinics of North America*, 1979, *26*, 565–579.

Brooks, J. G., Cotton, E. K., & Parry, W. H. Respiratory tract and mediastinum. In Kempe, C. H., (Ed.) *Current Pediatric Diagnosis and Treatment*, 5th ed. Los Altos, California: Lange Medical Publications, 1978, pp. 269–320.

Gephart, H. R. Minor acute illnesses of childhood. In Leitch, C. J., & Tinker, R. V. (Eds.). *Primary Care*. Philadelphia: F. A. Davis, 1978, pp. 409–424.

Lumicao, G. G., & Heggie, A. D. Chlamydial infections. *The Pediatric Clinics of North America*, 1979, *26*, 269–282.

McMillan, J. A., Stockman, J. A., & Oski, F. A. *The Whole Pediatrician Catalog*. Volume 2. Philadelphia: W. B. Saunders, 1979.

Murray, H. W., and Tauzon, C. Atypical pneumonias. *The Medical Clinics of North America*, 1980, *64*, 507–527.

Nelson, W. E. *Textbook of pediatrics*, 11th ed. Philadelphia: W. B. Saunders, 1979.

Reichman, R. C., & Dolin, R. Viral pneumonias. *The Medical Clinics of North America*, 1980, *64*, 491–506.

Rytel, M. W., & Schlueter, D. P. Viral and mycoplasmal pneumonia. In Conn, H. F. (Ed.). *Current Therapy*. Philadelphia: W. B. Saunders, 1980, pp. 136–138.

Simkins, R. Croup and epiglottitis. *American Journal of Nursing*, 1981, *81*, 519–520.

Valmar, H. Respiratory infections in the older infant. *British Medical Journal*, 1980, *280*, 1438–1442.

CHAPTER **7**

HEART DISEASE

Judith Leavitt Devlin

Nurse practitioners screen for cardiovascular disease in infants and children primarily to detect congenital heart defects and acquired heart disease. Severe congenital defects are usually detected early since most of these infants are cyanotic, or have congestive heart failure, along with an abnormal physical exam. Asymptomatic defects are picked up during the routine physical exam when an organic murmur is heard. Acquired heart disease is most often a result of an untreated streptococcal infection that causes rheumatic heart disease. The nurse practitioner needs to detect and institute proper therapy early for streptococcal infections as well as refer children with organic murmurs to the pediatric cardiologist.

Heart murmurs in children frequently are heard during physical examination. Depending on the experience of the practitioner and the cooperation of the child, one may hear murmurs in up to 50% of all normal children at some time during their childhood (1). Yet, the incidence of congenital heart disease is about 6 to 7 per 1,000 live births, decreasing to about 3 per 1,000 by the age of 10 years (2). The development of a systematic approach to cardiac evaluation is therefore essential to the nurse practitioner in the primary care setting. It would not be cost effective to refer every child with a heart murmur to a pediatric cardiologist, nor would it be judicious, in terms of time, to overload subspecialists with normal children to evaluate. Thus, screening for organic heart disease rests with the professionals practicing in the primary care setting.

THE NORMAL HEART

FETAL CIRCULATION

The heart begins developing in the third week of embryonic life. Initially, the heart is a tube-like structure that receives blood into one end and pumps it out the other. By the eighth, or tenth week of fetal life, this tube has transformed into a structure able to sustain growing fetal life and is capable of rapidly changing at birth to sustain independent circulation. Understandably, most congenital anomalies begin during the first 10 weeks of life.

Fetal circulation differs from extrauterine circulation since oxygenation occurs at the placenta rather than in the lungs. Blood is oxygenated by the mother and travels to the fetus via the placenta. Blood from the placenta flows to the fetal liver through the umbilical vein. Part of this oxygenated blood flows directly into the hepatic circulation, and part shunts through the vessel connecting the liver and the inferior vena cava (ductus venosus). Blood then flows through the inferior vena cava into the right atrium. Unoxygenated blood from the lower extremities also enters the right atrium through the inferior vena cava, making a mixture of oxygenated and unoxygenated blood. However, the blood is still highly oxygenated at this point.

This highly oxygenated inferior vena cava blood then flows to the left atrium, bypassing the right ventricle and lungs, via the foramen ovale, a structure that permits only right to left flow. In addition, a small amount of blood from the pulmonary veins enters the left atrium. Blood flows from the left atrium to the left ventricle, then out to the aorta. From here the mixed, but highly oxygenated blood flows through the coronary and cerebral arteries.

The superior vena cava brings unoxygenated blood from the head, upper extremities and heart. Blood from this source flows into the right atrium then into the right ventricle, rather than to the left atrium, and into the pulmonary artery. From the pulmonary artery, blood flows in two directions: a small amount flows to the lungs, and the larger amount flows to the aorta through the ductus arteriosus, the fetal connection between the pulmonary artery and the aorta. The blood in the aorta mixes with some of the blood ejected from the left ventricle. This highly unoxygenated blood flows to the lower extremities, then returns to the placenta via the umbilical arteries for oxygenation.

CHANGES AT BIRTH

At birth, the clamping and cutting of the cord, along with lung expansion, causes rapid changes in fetal circulation allowing the neonate to oxygenate independent of the placenta. Cessation of blood through the umbilical vein eliminates flow through the ductus venosus which rapidly undergoes thrombosis, rendering total occlusion of the passageway.

Since the lungs are not used to oxygenate the fetus, the pulmonary vessels are constricted to create a high pressure and to prevent blood flow into the pulmonary vasculature in utero. When the neonate takes the first breath of air and expands the alveoli, this pressure decreases creating a higher pressure in the left atrium that closes the foramen ovale. If the foramen ovale fails to close, the neonate will have a form of atrial septal defect.

The pressure in the lungs does not decrease to a normal level until 4 to 6 weeks of age. During this time, the right ventricle pumps more forcefully to get blood into the pulmonary vessels. The pressure in the right ventricle is equal to that in the left ventricle until the pulmonary pressure decreases. If the neonate has a ventricular spetal defect (VSD), the turbulence of blood and murmur will not be heard since there is no pressure difference between the chambers. Infants with large VSDs may develop congestive heart failure, while those with small defects usually have only an abnormal murmur at 4 to 6 weeks of age.

Finally, the rise in oxygen in the blood stimulates constriction of the ductus arteriosis. If the ductus does not close, the neonate has a patent ductus arteriosus (PDA).

Blood flows through the independent circulatory system as follows: unoxygenated blood returns to the right atrium via the superior and inferior vena cava; blood in the right atrium flows into the right ventricle through the tricuspid valve; blood is ejected through the pulmonary valve into the pulmonary arteries to the lungs, where blood is oxygenated and returned to the left atrium via the pulmonary veins. Blood then flows through the bicuspid or mitral valve into the left ventricle, then through the aortic valve into the aorta; the oxygenated blood flows to the entire body, returning to the right atrium to repeat the cycle.

SYSTOLE AND DIASTOLE

The sequence of events in the heart is divided into two phases: systole and diastole. During systole, the ventricles contract, forcing blood into the pulmonary artery and the aorta. If either of these valves are stenotic or narrowed, there will be a greater turbulence of blood as it is ejected through these valves. Therefore, in systole, one hears the murmurs of pulmonic and aortic stenosis. Also, at the onset of systole, the bicuspid and tricuspid valves snap shut. If either of these two valves is incompetent and allows a backflow of blood into the respective atrium, the murmur produced will be heard in systole.

During diastole the heart relaxes. At the onset of diastole, the bicuspid and mitral valves open as blood flows passively into the ventricles. If either of these two valves is stenotic, again a turbulence of blood will produce a murmur. Conversely, if either the pulmonic or aortic valves allows a backflow of blood, a murmur will be heard.

HEART SOUNDS

The basic heart sounds include the first (S_1), the second (S_2), the third (S_3) and the fourth (S_4). S_1 represents the onset of systole or closing of the tricuspid and mitral valves. S_2 is the onset of diastole or closing of the aortic and pulmonic valves.

S_1 is heard loudest at the apex. Although it is normally split, the splitting is rarely detected in the tricuspid area when the tricuspid component is audible. What appears to be a split S_1, heard at the apex, is usually an S_4, or a systolic click, rather than a split S_1. S_4 is a low pitched sound which is best heard with the bell. Systolic clicks are high pitched sounds which are best heard with the diaphragm. Systolic clicks are associated with aortic and pulmonic stenosis.

S_2 is loudest at the aortic and pulmonic areas since it is generated from the closure of the aortic and pulmonic valves. The first component of S_2 is closure of the aortic valve, which closes first since the left ventricle depolarizes and contracts slightly before the right ventricle. The second component of S_2 is the pulmonic valve closure. To accentuate the normal split of S_2, concentrate on the sound in the pulmonic area where the second component is most intense. Listen carefully for changes during inspiration. Normally, the time between closure of the aortic and pulmonic valves is increased during inspiration. During inspiration, the intrathoracic pressure decreases, allowing more blood to return to the right atrium. The increased amount of blood to the right heart takes longer to flow, making closure of the pulmonic valve later than during expiration. S_2 should always vary with respirations. A wide and fixed split is associated with an atrial septal defect and should be referred to the pediatric cardiologist.

S_3 and S_4 represent the sounds made during diastolic filling. Children and young adults can normally have a third heart sound, but rarely a normal fourth heart sound. A fourth heart sound in children usually indicates that the right atrium has an increased pressure and/or volume that is, an atrial septal defect, whereas an S_4 in adolescents usually indicates congestive heart failure.

EVALUATION

HISTORY

The value of a thorough history cannot be overemphasized in screening for congenital anomalies. It is the first step in differentiating the innocent from the organic murmur. Areas that should be included in the history are reviewed here.

Gestational History

The importance of the gestational history is to determine exposure to rubella, teratogenic agents, and excessive maternal alcohol use. A positive history in any three of these situations supports a suspicion of a congenital anomaly.

Past Health

The practitioner needs to rule out a past history of cardiac symptoms in the infant or child. Signs of cardiac disease include cyanosis, dyspnea, poor feeding, tachypnea, and poor growth rate. In the older child, inquire about a past history of rheumatic fever or prolonged illness that may have been untreated.

Family History

Familial occurrence of congenital heart disease is uncommon. However, the risk of developing heart disease is 10 times greater for an infant if there is a positive family history.

Personal/Social History

It is important to establish the child's activity level, exercise tolerance, and progress in school in order to differentiate the normal child from the child with cardiac disease. Asking children if they are able to keep up with their peers is a good screening question.

General

The general health and the parents' perception of their child's health gives the practitioner the overall picture that leads to other avenues of investigation. Early congestive heart failure in the infant can present as vaguely as poor sucking and poor growth rate. Other general signs of cardiac disease include restlessness, irritability, and diaphoresis.

Respiratory

Tachypnea, dyspnea, wheezing, and grunting in infancy are all abnormal and suggestive of heart disease. In addition, children with cardiac disease are more apt to have frequent lower respiratory tract infections.

Cardiovascular

The following signs and symptoms indicate cardiac disease: cyanosis that can be peripheral or central, constant or intermittent, that is, only with crying or feeding, when oxygen demands are higher; squatting, which is the hallmark of tetralogy of Fallot; syncope and chest pain, which are symptoms of aortic stenosis. Edema is not associated with cardiac disease in children, yet does suggest renal disease.

PHYSICAL EXAMINATION

The cardiovascular examination is as important as the medical history when screening for congenital heart disease. The exam is presented here, followed by descriptions of the four most common innocent murmurs. Screening for congenital heart disease is a manageable problem once the normal heart sounds are recognized by the examiner. The generalist can then recognize an innocent murmur confidently, and refer those of organic nature. Moreover, the generalist avoids the confusion of every organic possibility, leaving that to the pediatric cardiologist.

General Inspection

Evaluate body size and any distress in the infant or child. Observe the child for activity level and body posture, that is, squatting.

Height and Weight

Graph height and weight on percentile graphs to insure that the child does not deviate from the growth curve. Poor growth may be present in children with congenital heart disease.

Temperature

Remember that an elevated temperature will accentuate an innocent murmur because of the higher blood volume flowing through the heart valves. Any murmur heard during a febrile illness should be rechecked once the fever has resolved.

Pulse

The easiest and most accurate pulse in the infant or child is the apical pulse. Evaluate the pulse for rate and rhythm (see Table 7.1 for average heart rates in infants and children at rest). The heart rhythm is usually regular in children, although it is not uncommon to note changes with respiration, a normal variation known as sinus arrythmia. In sinus arrythmia, the heart accelerates with inspiration and slows with expiration.

Respiration

Observe respiration for rate and pattern. The rate varies greatly in infants and children, depending on exercise, emotion, and the presence of illness. The respiratory rate in the newborn ranges from 30 to 80 per minute, in early childhood between 20 and 40 per minute, and in late childhood between 15 and 25. At age 15, the respiratory rate reaches the adult range. Next, observe the pattern of the respirations. The newborn pattern can normally vary from rapid breathing to periods of apnea and should be observed for a full minute to determine true rate.

Blood Pressure

Taking the blood pressure is perhaps the most overlooked vital sign in pediatrics. One assumes the value will be inaccurate and omits the procedure altogether to avoid the time-consuming task. However, most children over 3 years of age will be very cooperative once they understand the procedure. It will be difficult to obtain a blood pressure on a child who is anxious, crying, or uncooperative. The procedure can be done at the end of the exam or on a subsequent visit. All children should have their blood pressure evaluated at both upper and lower extremities at least once before entering school to screen for coarctation of the aorta (also see peripheral pulses). Moreover, children 3 years and over should have their blood pressure measured yearly as part of health maintenance care.

Blood pressure can be taken in infants and children using one of three techniques. The first is with the sphygmomanometer and the procedure is the same as that used in adults. The width of the blood pressure cuff should be one-half the width of the upper extremity. The bladder, or inflatable rub-

Table 7.1. Average Heart Rate of Infants and Children At Rest

Age	Average Rate	Two-Standard Deviations
Birth	140	50
1st 6 months	130	50
6–12 months	115	40
1–2 years	110	40
2–6 years	103	35
6–10 years	95	30
10–14 years	95	30

Reproduced with permission from Bates, Barbara, *A Guide to Physical Examination*, J. B. Lippincott Co., 1979.

ber bag, should go around the entire extremity. Proper cuff size is important since a cuff too small falsely elevates the blood pressure and a cuff too large may falsely lower the blood pressure and cover the brachial artery in the antecubital space. The fourth Korotkoff sound, or the muffling sound, is usually absent in children, so the fifth sound (or the disappearance of the sound) is used to denote diastolic blood pressure.

The second technique of ascertaining blood pressure is simply palpating a systolic pressure when the heart sounds are inaudible in the brachial artery. First, palpate the radial pulse. With the finger still on the pulse, pump up the cuff until the pulse is no longer felt. Finally, deflate the cuff approximately 2 to 4 mm Hg per second. The systolic pressure is the point at which the pulse is first felt. The diastolic pressure cannot be measured using the palpation method.

The third technique is the flush technique and gives a value between the systolic and diastolic pressures. Wrap the cuff around the arm, then elevate the extremity. While elevated, wrap an elastic bandage around the arm extending from the fingers to the antecubital space. Inflate the blood pressure cuff above the expected systolic pressure, then remove the bandage and lower the arm. Slowly decrease the cuff pressure until normal color returns to the extremity. At this point the value is recorded.

Normal blood pressures in children have been determined and can be monitored by using percentile charts (Figs. 7.1, 7.2). Any infant or child whose blood pressure is consistently greater than the 95th percentile should be referred for further evaluation.

Most children under 10 years of age with hypertension will have a secondary cause. The most common causes are renal disease (78%), renal arterial disease (12%), and coarctation of the aorta (2%) (3). In children over 10, a secondary cause of the hypertension is less likely. Depending on the study, the incidence of adolescent hypertension ranges from 1.4 to 11% (4). With

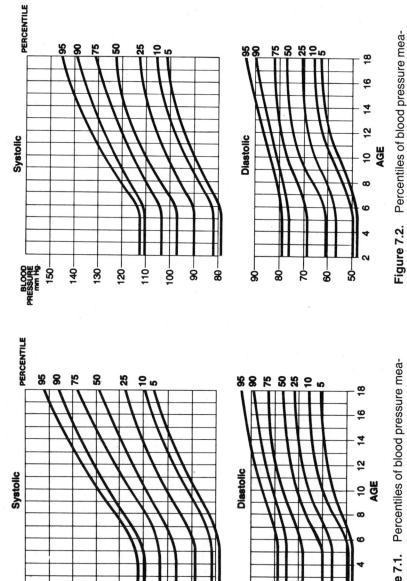

Figure 7.1. Percentiles of blood pressure measurement in boys (right arm, seated). (Source: PEDIATRICS 59, (5), Part 2, May, 1977.)

Figure 7.2. Percentiles of blood pressure measurement in girls (right arm, seated). (Source: PEDIATRICS 59, (5), Part 2, May, 1977.)

these data in mind, the need for blood pressure evaluation in this population is obvious.

Skin

Observe skin for pallor, cyanosis, and diaphoresis. Cyanosis may be more readily seen in the mucous membranes or circumoral region. Inspect the nail beds for cyanosis and clubbing.

HEENT

Observe the child for abnormal facies, that is, the classic facies of Down's syndrome, since approximately one half of all children with Down's syndrome have some type of congenital heart defect (5). Perform a funduscopic examination on children with an elevated blood pressure.

Thorax and Lungs

Assess the shape of the bony thorax for chest wall deformities. Children with a diminished anteroposterior diameter of the chest and an absence of the normal kyphosis of the thoracic spine usually have a Grade 1 to 3/6 systolic murmur in the pulmonic area. The organic-sounding murmur is actually quite innocent and called the "straight-back syndrome" (6). Assess breath sounds for character and adventitious sounds. Children with congestive heart failure usually have audible rales and wheezes.

Cardiovascular

A thorough cardiovascular examination involves both the heart and peripheral pulses. The peripheral pulses are frequently overlooked, but are essential when screening for cardiovascular disease.

Heart

The heart examination includes three of the four major components of the physical examination: inspection, palpation, and auscultation. Since percussing the heart does not give any more information to the examiner, it is omitted from the discussion.

Inspection. With the child supine, inspect the precordium for abnormal movement. Normally, the right and left precordial areas have symmetrical movements. Occasionally, the left precordium will be larger if the child has cardiomegaly.

Palpation. Palpate the precordium to determine the point of maximal impulse (PMI) and any abnormal pulsations, lifts, or heaves. Place the entire palmar surface of the hand across the lower sternum with the fingers extending across the left precordium. A heave felt with the heel of the hand indicates right ventricular hypertrophy; a heave felt with the finger pads indicates left ventricular hypertrophy. Heaves palpated in the right or left ventricular areas suggest enlarged chambers.

Next determine the PMI, or apical impulse. In children under 7 years, the PMI is located at the fourth left intercostal space just left of the midclavicular line. In children over 7 years, the PMI is normally at the fifth left intercostal space. If the right ventricle is enlarged, the PMI displaces laterally. If the left ventricle is enlarged the PMI displaces both laterally and downward. In addition, a diffuse PMI indicates left ventricular hypertrophy.

Completely palpate in each of the following areas for abnormal pulsations: aortic, pulmonic, right ventricular, left ventricular, and epigastric. Accentuated pulsations in the aortic area (second intercostal space to the right of the sternum) are not usually seen in children with or without heart disease. A palpable thrill in this area sometimes accompanies aortic stenosis. An abnormal pulsation in the pulmonic area (second intercostal space to the left of the sternum) is due to an increase in pressure or flow to the pulmonary artery, as in pulmonic stenosis. A thrill in the pulmonary area is also associated with pulmonary stenosis. A thrill palpated in the right ventricular area may be felt in infants and children with a ventricular septal defect; the thrill, sometimes associated with mitral stenosis, can be palpated in the left ventricular area. An abnormal increase of the aortic pulse in the epigastric area is associated with aortic regurgitation.

Auscultation. Auscultation of the heart includes evaluation of the heart rate and rhythm, the heart sounds, and the presence or absence of any heart murmurs. One listens with both the diaphragm and the bell of the stethoscope. The diaphragm picks up the higher pitched sounds, such as systolic ejection murmurs, diastolic murmurs of aortic and pulmonary regurgitation, and pericardial friction rubs. The bell picks up such low pitched sounds as gallops, and the diastolic murmurs of mitral, and tricuspid stenosis.

Initially, listen to the rate and rhythm. Count the pulse for 15 seconds and multiply by four if the rhythm is regular. Count for 60 seconds if the rhythm is irregular. If irregular, determine if the rhythm varies with respirations as in sinus arrhythmia, has a pattern to the irregularity, or is totally irregular.

Next, listen to each of the ausculatory areas in the following order: aortic, pulmonic, tricuspid, and mitral. In each area identify S_1 and S_2. Remember, S_1 should be louder at the apex and S_2 should be louder at the aortic and pulmonic areas.

Listen closely to S_2 in the pulmonic area to differentiate physiologic splitting from an abnormally wide split that does not vary with respirations. Determine if S_3 and S_4 are present, remembering that they are heard in diastole. S_3 mimicks the sounds made when one says "Ken-túck-y" aloud and S_4 when one says "Ténn-e-see."

Now concentrate on only systole in each area. Determine the presence or absence of a systolic murmur. If present, describe it using the following descriptors:

1. Timing—early, mid, or late systole; all of systole (holosystolic)
2. Location—where the murmur is most intense and radiation to other areas
3. Intensity, graded 1 to 6
   Grade 1: faint, not heard in all positions, usually only heard by the cardiologist
   Grade 2: quiet and heard in all positions
   Grade 3: louder than 2, not associated with a thrill
   Grade 4: loud and associated with a thrill
   Grade 5: loud enough to be heard with the stethoscope off the chest; associated with a thrill
   Grade 6: so loud the murmur is heard with the stethoscope off the chest; associated with a thrill
4. Pitch—high, medium, or low
5. Quality—soft or blowing, harsh, vibratory, or rumbling.

Next, concentrate only on diastole in each area. Describe any murmurs heard using the above criteria. A diastolic murmur is always abnormal and should be referred to a pediatric cardiologist for further evaluation.

Finally, listen for sounds that have both a systolic and diastolic component. The venous hum, an innocent murmur described in the next section, is a continuous (both systolic and diastolic) murmur heard in the supraclavicular areas. Differentiate the venous hum from the continuous murmur of a patent ductus arteriosus, which is heard best beneath the left clavicle and is louder during systole.

A pericardial friction rub also has both systolic and diastolic components. It is best described as a grating sound and can be mimicked by rubbing hair together next to one's ear canal. Pericardial friction rubs are always abnormal and may be present in life-threatening conditions, so such patients should always be referred.

Peripheral Pulses

No cardiovascular examination is complete without careful assessment of the peripheral pulses. The examiner should palpate the radial, brachial, femoral, posterior tibial, and dorsalis pedis pulses. Palpate the pulse bilaterally and compare the volume for equality. Use the following classifications:

0 - absent
1 - diminished
2 - normal
3 - fuller than 3, but normal
4 - bounding

Absent or delayed femoral pulses are indicative of coarctation of the aorta. In addition, the child may have accentuated pulses and elevated blood pressures in the upper extremities, along with a decreased blood pressure in the legs.

An infant or child with bounding peripheral pulses may have a patent ductus arteriosus. If in doubt, return to auscultation for reevaluation.

Abdominal Examination

The abdominal examination plays a part in screening for cardiovascular diseases by helping the practitioner rule out congestive heart failure. Normally, the edge of the infant's liver may be palpated 2 cms below the right costal margin. An engorged liver, along with other signs and symptoms of congestive heart failure, should be referred immediately to a pediatric cardiologist. The spleen is not usually palpable unless infection is present. However, the tip may be palpable in healthy children.

TYPES OF INNOCENT MURMURS

When an examiner hears a cardiac murmur, he/she must decide whether it is normal or abnormal. There are several general characteristics of all innocent murmurs:

1. Innocent murmurs are always systolic. Any diastolic murmur is considered organic.
2. Innocent murmurs are Grade 1 to Grade 3. If the examiner palpates a thrill, the murmur can be considered organic.

3. Innocent murmurs are not associated with cardiac symptoms, for example, dyspnea or cyanosis.
4. Innocent murmurs are associated with normal heart sounds.
5. Innocent murmurs usually do not radiate.

Specific types of innocent murmurs are commonly heard in primary care settings. Each will be described here and will include criteria for differential diagnosis.

VIBRATORY MURMUR

The most common type of innocent murmur is the vibratory murmur. It is usually Grade 1-3, medium pitched, mid-systolic and heard best along the lower left sternal border without radiation. One must rule out the murmur of a ventricular septic defect, which usually has a harsh quality and may radiate to other areas of the chest.

PULMONARY FLOW MURMUR

This murmur is also midsystolic, with a soft, medium pitch, but is located along the upper left sternal border. Most authorities believe that the etiology of the sound is a turbulent blood flow through the right ventricular outflow tract. The murmur of an atrial septal defect may sound like the pulmonary flow murmur and it can be differentiated by the splitting of the second heart sound. An atrial septal defect produces a second heart sound that is widely split and does not vary with respirations.

VENOUS HUM

The venous hum is a continuous murmur heard in systole and diastole. It can be heard in the right and left supraclavicular fossa, although it is more commonly heard on the right. The sound is thought to be caused by the turbulence of blood in the jugular veins. It is accentuated in a child in the sitting position. The murmur will decrease or disappear entirely when the child is supine or the examiner applies pressure to the jugular veins. The venous hum may be confused with the continuous murmur of a patent ductus arteriosus. However, the ductus murmur will not vary with position and is heard best beneath the left clavicle.

ARTERIAL BRUIT

The arterial bruit is sometimes referred to as a systolic ejection murmur. It is heard over the carotid artery in most children, as the sound originates from the carotid artery bifurcation. The examiner who hears the arterial bruit must differentiate it from the murmur of aortic stenosis that can radiate to the neck.

MANAGEMENT OF CARDIAC MURMURS

A child with a clear, innocent cardiac murmur needs no special follow-up. However, the murmur should be recorded in the permanent record and the child seen at routine intervals.

REFERRAL

The child with a murmur that is equivocal, presents a perplexing problem. Depending on the experience of the practitioner, one of two decisions can be made. The practitioner can obtain a chest x-ray film and ECG and if those two tests are normal, he or she can be reassured that the child does not have an organic murmur. The second option is to refer the child to the pediatric cardiologist. This author believes that the latter choice is not as good since the incidence of innocent murmurs is so high that the cardiologists can find themselves overloaded with innocent murmurs to evaluate.

If the nurse practitioner hears an unequivocally abnormal murmur, the child needs to be referred to the pediatric cardiologist. A child who has cyanosis or symptoms of congestive heart failure should be referred immediately for further evaluation.

COUNSELING

This author believes that parents should always be informed about a child's innocent murmur. It is the practitioner's responsibility to explain the terms of the innocent or functional murmur thoroughly so that the parents do not leave believing that their child has heart disease. Moreover, if a murmur is heard later in the child's life during a febrile illness, the parents can inform the examiner that normal murmurs have been heard before and thus aid in the evaluation process.

Parents of children with suspicious or clearly organic murmurs should be prepared for the possibility of further evaluation by the pediatric cardiologist.

RHEUMATIC FEVER

Rheumatic fever is a systemic inflammatory disease that results from an untreated streptococcal infection. The prevalence is about 1 per 1,000 in school-age children (7). Rheumatic fever affects the heart in approximately one-third to one-half of all cases (8).

HISTORY AND PHYSICAL EXAMINATION

The child with rheumatic fever appears with various symptoms. Early symptoms of malaise and fever are common. In addition, the child may have arthritis with red, swollen, tender joints that lasts approximately three weeks. Usually, the larger weight-bearing joints are affected, although the shoulders, wrists, and small joints in the hand can be involved. Arthritis is a major criterion of the disease and must be differentiated from arthralgia, a minor criterion (see Table 7.2). Pericarditis may cause the child to have chest pain, a low-grade fever, tachycardia, a pericardial friction rub, and an elevated sedimentation rate. The child frequently develops a skin rash in the acute phase of the disease. Although they may go unnoticed subcutaneous nodules may be present. Parents may report a change in behavior, that is,

Table 7.2. Jones Criteria

Major Manifestations
Carditis
Polyarthritis
Chorea
Erythema marginatum
Subcutaneous nodules
Minor Manifestations
Positive history of rheumatic fever or rheumatic heart disease
Arthralgia
Fever
Elevated sedimentation rate
Positive reactive protein
Leukocytosis
Prolonged P–R interval

emotional lability or sudden involuntary movements in the child. The examiner needs to rule out Sydenham's chorea, which is characterized by brief, involuntary movements of muscles in the face, a limb, or one side of the body.

The cardiac examination is frequently abnormal in rheumatic fever. During the acute phase of the disease, the heart valves may become edematous and more vulnerable to vegetation collection. The mitral and aortic valves are most vulnerable since they close with the highest pressure. The tricuspid and pulmonic valves close with markedly less pressure and are less apt to become diseased. The typical murmurs heard are mitral and aortic insufficiency. The murmur of aortic insufficiency is heard in diastole and should not be confused with an innocent murmur. The murmur of mitral insufficiency, however, is heard in systole. One differentiates the murmur of mitral insufficiency from an innocent murmur by listening closely to timing. This murmur is holosystolic, heard best at the apex, and may radiate to the left axilla. No innocent murmurs have these characteristics.

DIAGNOSTIC TESTS

The diagnosis of rheumatic fever is made by using the Jones criteria (see Table 7.2). Rheumatic fever is suspected when two major, or one major and two minor criteria are present with evidence of a prior streptococcal infection (9).

MANAGEMENT

Counseling

Rheumatic fever is treated with bed rest, penicillin, and aspirin. The child needs to remain in bed during the acute phase of the illness to decrease heart workload. As the sedimentation rate returns to normal, the child's activity can be resumed.

Pharmacology

Penicillin is given in doses of 0.5 to 1.0 million units daily in divided doses for 10 to 14 days. Aspirin is given in doses of 170 mg/kg/day initially and reduced to 60 mg/kg/day after 3 days. Steroid therapy should not be instituted since it can increase the likelihood of a relapse of the carditis.

Prophylaxis

Rheumatic fever prophylaxis is recommended until the age of 20, or until five years after the last attack. The drug of choice is oral penicillin V, 125 mg twice daily. If compliance is low, 1.2 million units of benzathine penicillin can be given intramuscularly each month.

STUDY QUESTIONS

Circle all that apply.

1. Johnny Jones is a 4-year-old boy who you have been following for the past three years. He has had an unremarkable history except for the usual communicable diseases. He is in the clinic for a routine health maintenance visit. On physical examination, you hear a Grade 2/6, soft midsystolic murmur along the lower left sternal border. The murmur does not radiate. The most likely diagnosis is:

   a. ventricular septal defect
   b. pulmonary flow murmur
   c. vibratory murmur
   d. aortic stenosis

2. Which characteristics would make you suspect an organic murmur?

   a. harsh quality
   b. radiation to other areas of the chest
   c. PMI at the fourth left ICS, 2 cms beyond the midclavicular line
   d. Grade 3/6

3. You see a 5-week-old infant for the first time since he was examined in the newborn nursery. The mother reports that he is "not a very good eater" and seems to breathe "heavy." To confirm your suspicion of congestive heart failure, you ask the following questions:

   a. Does he have frequent diarrhea?
   b. How long does it take for him to finish a 3 to 4 ounce bottle?
   c. Does he need to stop sucking frequently to "catch his breath?"
   d. Are respirations irregular?

4. Which of the following questions would probably *not* be helpful in differentiating the normal infant from the infant with congestive heart failure?

    a. Is there a family history of congenital heart defects?

    b. Does the child look swollen around his eyes after a period of sleep?

    c. Does the infant turn blue when he cries?

    d. Does the child become diaphoretic when he feeds?

5. If the foramen ovale fails to close, the child has which of the following conditions?

    a. patent ductus arteriosus

    b. atrial septal defect

    c. ventricular septal defect

    d. aortic stenosis

6. The following is/are true of a VSD murmur:

    a. it can be detected in the newborn nursery

    b. it resembles a venous hum

    c. it usually has a harsh quality

    d. it can radiate to the entire precordium

7. A heart murmur is caused by which of the following events?

    a. narrowing of a heart valve

    b. leakage of a heart valve

    c. turbulence of blood

    d. heart failure

8. The first heart sound is heard best (most intense) in which area?

    a. apex

    b. second ICS to the left of the sternum

    c. second ICS to the right of the sternum

    d. along the left sternal border

9. The splitting of the second heart sound is heard best in which ausculatory areas?

    a. aortic

    b. pulmonic

    c. tricuspid

    d. mitral

10. A wide, fixed splitting of the second heart sound is diagnostic of which congenital heart defect?

    a. tetralogy of Fallot

    b. pulmonic stenosis

   c. atrial septal defect
   d. is normal

11. Which valves close during diastole?

   a. mitral and tricuspid
   b. mitral and aortic
   c. aortic and pulmonic
   d. aortic and tricuspid

12. The murmur of aortic stenosis is heard during which cardiac cycle?

   a. systole only
   b. diastole only
   c. both systole and diastole

13. The following statement is true about S_3:

   a. it is normal in children and adults
   b. it is one of the sounds made during passive ventricular filling
   c. it is always abnormal
   d. it is the sound made during systole

14. Which of the following murmurs are most common in rheumatic heart disease?

   a. mitral stenosis
   b. pulmonic insufficiency
   c. aortic regurgitation
   d. mitral regurgitation

15. Which of the following symptoms are not common in rheumatic fever?

   a. fever
   b. erythema marginatum
   c. chest pain
   d. nausea

ANSWERS

1. c   4. b
2. a, b, c, d   5. b
3. a   6. c and d

7. a, b, c   12. a
8. a   13. b
9. b   14. c
10. c   15. a, b, c
11. c

REFERENCES

1. Carne, S. *Pediatric Care—Child Health in Family Practice*. Philadelphia: Lippincott, 1976.
2. Sapire, D. W. Innocent murmurs in children—an everpresent problem in practice. *Primary Care,* 1974, *1,* 221–232.
3. Bates, B. *A guide to physical examination,* 2nd ed. Philadelphia: Lippincott, 1979.
4. Loggie, J. Essential hypertension in adolescents. *Post Graduate Medicine,* 1974, *56, 6,* 134.
5. Nora, J. J. & Nora, A. H. The evolution of specific genetic and environmental counseling in congenital heart diseases. *Circulation,* 1978, *57,* 205–213.
6. Nudel, D. B. & Gootman, N. Functional murmurs in children. *New York State Journal of Medicine,* 1978, *78,* 2070–2072.
7. deCastro, F. J. & Rolfe, U. T. *The pediatric nurse practitioner.* St. Louis: C. V. Mosby, 1972.
8. *Primer on the rheumatic disease,* 7th ed, 74, 1973.
9. Silverman, M. E. *Examination of the heart, part one: data collection—the clinical history.* New York: American Heart Association, 1973.

CHAPTER 8

GASTROINTESTINAL PROBLEMS

Lucinda L. Carlson

Pediatric problems involving the gastrointestinal (GI) tract account for a large percentage of office visits. Problems run the full spectrum, from benign feeding problems to surgical emergencies like appendicitis. Diagnosis may be complicated by second- or third-party histories that are often incomplete or unreliable, and by a patient population that is frequently uncooperative during examination. Thorough history and examination, as well as an awareness of the numerous causes of gastrointestinal problems, will help untangle the many puzzles presented daily. A five area overview (abdominal pain, vomiting, diarrhea, constipation, and parasites) will be presented in this chapter, with several disease entities considered in each area.

ABDOMINAL PAIN

APPENDICITIS

Appendicitis is rare before 2 years of age and unusual before 5, with the frequency increasing as a child gets older, to a peak in teenage and early adult years. A seasonal increase of incidents in autumn and spring is also noted. It is the most common condition requiring intraabdominal surgery in childhood. Appendicitis in the young child is atypical and the disease course rapid, so that the appendices of children under 4 years old usually have ruptured before the child is seen by a health provider.

History and Physical Examination

The classic triad of symptoms found in the adult, that of persistent right lower quadrant (RLQ) pain, localized abdominal tenderness and rigidity, and slight fever, is strongly suggestive of appendicitis in the child also. Unfortunately, such a clear picture is uncommon in children. Abdominal pain followed by fever and vomiting are usually the presenting symptoms in older children, but vomiting as a primary symptom, even before abdominal pain begins, is not uncommon in young children and infants. Vomiting, irritability, listlessness, pallor, anorexia, and fever are more typical symptoms in the young child.

The abdominal pain, usually beginning in the periumbilical area, and then localizing in the RLQ (McBurney's point), is constant, severe, and aggravated by cough or movement. Because of the peritoneal irritation involved, the child may limp, double up, or refrain from all activity in an effort to prevent pain. An infant may lie quietly with legs drawn up to ease abdominal pain. Duration of the pain is important since severe abdominal pain of more than six hours is unlikely to be simple gastroenteritis. Persistent RLQ tenderness, especially with involuntary abdominal muscle spasm and guarding, is one of the most reliable signs of appendicitis in a child. Eliciting RLQ pain with a cough or gentle shaking of an infant's thigh can be helpful corollaries in attempting to establish a positive psoas sign. Rebound tenderness is not so reliable in young children because of feces and air in the cecum.

Constipation occurs in older children but, due to the rapidity of the disease in young children, diarrhea may be present. Leukocytosis and increased pulse rate may occur. A rectal exam is indicated; one should check for right-sided tenderness and possibly a mass, if the appendix has ruptured.

Diagnostic Tests

A CBC shows mild leukocytosis—rarely more than 15,000/cu mm. A flat plate x-ray film of the abdomen may show a fecalith in the lumen of the appendix. If diagnosis is questionable, other lab studies are used to rule out various conditions that may mimic an acute abdomen, (e.g., gastroenteritis, urinary tract infection (UTI), mesenteric adenitis, pneumonia).

Management

Definitive diagnosis and treatment can only be done surgically with appendectomy. If appendicitis is suspected, rapid referral for immediate surgical consultation is indicated.

INTUSSUSCEPTION

Intussusception is the most common cause of intestinal obstruction in the first three years of life. It is rare under 3 months of age and decreases in frequency after 36 months. It is three times more common in boys and also shows a seasonal spring-fall pattern. In most cases, the upper portion of the bowel, usually at a point immediately proximal to the ileocecal valve, invaginates into the lower segment of the bowel, resulting in an ileocolic type of intussusception. The impaired venous return causes bowel swelling, hemorrhage, incarceration with necrosis and eventual perforation, peritonitis, gangrene, and shock if untreated. Although some intussusceptions will spontaneously reduce, most will result in death if untreated.

History

Typically, a previously healthy infant between 3 and 12 months suddenly develops violent, intermittent, paroxysmal periods of abdominal pain with screaming and drawing up of the legs. The attacks may last from 5 to 30 minutes. The period between attacks may vary. The infant appears quite ill, pale, and lethargic. Although the infant may initially play between attacks, as time goes on, he or she becomes progressively weaker and more "shocky." Vomiting soon follows and bloody bowel movements appear within 12 hours ("currant jelly stools").

Physical Examination

Severe prostration and fever are noted. Abdomen is tender and may be distended. On palpation, a sausage-shaped mass, usually in the right upper quadrant, can be found in the early stages. Presence of bloody mucus with rectal examination supports the diagnosis.

Diagnostic Tests

Barium enema is needed for definitive diagnosis and may also reduce the intussusception.

Management

Intussusception constitutes an abdominal emergency and requires immediate referral for medical or surgical reduction.

MESENTERIC LYMPHADENITIS

Mesenteric lymphadenitis is a common cause of abdominal pain in childhood. Generally, the only time it causes problems is when it mimics an acute appendicitis.

History

Typically, abdominal pain begins after an upper respiratory infection. The pain starts in the right lower quadrant, but is not persistent and may be found in any part of the abdomen. Fever can be significant; vomiting is not.

Physical Examination

Abdominal tenderness following the route of the mesentery (from McBurney's point to left of the umbilicus) may be present. Pain may shift as the client is rolled from side to side. Enlarged mesenteric glands may be palpable in the right lower quadrant.

Diagnostic Tests

Lab tests are used to rule out other diseases since no specific test for mesenteric lymphadenitis exists. Leukocytosis is usually higher than in appendicitis, with elevations greater than 20,000 WBC/cu mm frequently found.

Management

Only supportive care and symptomatic treatment is needed as the disease is self-limiting.

INGUINAL HERNIA

An inguinal hernia may be present at birth or may manifest itself at nearly any age. Most are of the indirect type, with boys affected nine times as often as girls. If incarceration of the hernia occurs, it is usually in the first ten months of life and more common in girls.

History

Uncomplicated inguinal hernias rarely cause pain. A history of inguinal fullness with coughing or after long standing may be given. A hernia usually will reduce itself spontaneously when an infant relaxes or an older child lies down. A loop of bowel that has herniated may become partially obstructed or incarcerated, leading to pain, irritability, and symptoms of intestinal obstruction, (i.e., distension and bilious vomiting). In girls, the ovary is the most likely organ to herniate.

Physical Examination

On inspection and palpation of the inguinal areas, a characteristic bulging or mass may be noted, especially with increased abdominal pressure caused by crying or bearing down. A herniated ovary is palpable as an almond-sized, moveable nodule. If the bowel has herniated and strangulated, redness, swelling, and tenderness is present.

Diagnosis

The diagnosis of inguinal hernia is made by history and physical examination alone. In early childhood, an accurate description of the swelling by a competent observer generally is sufficient for diagnosis.

Management

Since treatment in all cases is surgical repair, referral is indicated. Any inguinal hernia that cannot be reduced requires immediate surgical attention. Resection of the bowel may be required, if strangulation has occurred.

RECURRENT ABDOMINAL PAIN

Recurrent abdominal pain (RAP) affects approximately 10% of the pediatric population. Onset is around 5 to 10 years of age in boys and 8 to 12 years in girls. Incidence of RAP is slightly higher in girls. By one broad definition, a child is said to have recurrent abdominal pain if at least three episodes of pain severe enough to affect activities have been experienced over a period longer than three months. In approximately 50% of cases, the pain occurs more than once a week. The disease has a strong psychosomatic basis which is reflected in the personality characteristics of the affected children. Poor self-image, inability to relate to peers, immaturity, dependence, and impulsivity are often noted. The diagnosis is based on the history, absence of organic disease, and presence of a psychologic/emotional problem in the child or family.

History

Periumbilical or epigastric pain is experienced in recurrent attacks which vary in length from minutes to several days, though usually lasting about an hour. The pain bears no relationship to foods, eating, bowel movements, time of day, activity, or medicines. (If the pain consistently occurs when the child is getting ready for school, an alternate diagnosis of "school phobia" should be suspected.) Descriptions of the pain are inconsistent, varying from sharp to dull. Vomiting, nausea, headache, and pallor may accompany the pain. School or social events, illness or instability in the home, and other exciting or stressful occurrences can precipitate or exacerbate the abdominal pain. Concomitant emotional disturbances with poor school performance, enuresis, phobias, and sleeping problems are common. The family history frequently reveals other members with similar abdominal problems.

Physical Examination

A thorough examination is essential although results are usually normal. Mild, diffuse abdominal tenderness may be present.

Diagnostic Tests

A complete blood cell count (CBC) and sedimentation rate, urinalysis and urine culture, and stool for occult blood usually are sufficient to rule out organic disease. Gallbladder and gastrointestinal series may be indicated if symptomatology is atypical. A dilemma exists as to how many lab tests to perform when a psychosomatic illness is strongly suspected.

Management

Treatment consists of education and reassurance of the parents and the child. Explanation of the emotional basis is important but may be difficult for some parents to accept. Since the pain is real to the child, a sympathetic approach is needed. Medications are to be avoided. An immediate return to school is advised, giving the child a "face-saving" reason if a large amount of school has been missed. In 75 to 80% of clients, the symptoms will resolve with time, although 50% can expect some reoccurrence. Psychologic/psychiatric referral may be needed in as many as 20% of the cases.

VOMITING

FEEDING PROBLEMS AND REGURGITATION

Regurgitation is common in infants up to 9 months old and is no cause for concern if the infant is growing well and has no other symptoms. Faulty feeding techniques are the most common cause of significant regurgitation in the infant.

History

Close questioning about feeding techniques and the type and amount of food eaten often will reveal the underlying problem(s). Infrequent burping, allowing too much air into the nipple, improper positioning, overfeeding, overstimulation during feeding, or the infant's taking too much too quickly all may cause an inordinate amount of regurgitation. The "vomiting" will not be forceful and is usually in small amounts. If a child eats when overtired, overexcited, angry, or frightened he or she also may have difficulty digesting food, resulting in vomiting of the undigested stomach contents.

Physical Examination

Physical examination is normal and the infant is healthy and growing.

Diagnostic Tests

Diagnosis is made from history and examination alone. No laboratory tests are needed if other symptoms are absent.

Management

Treatment consists of correction of improper feeding techniques and reassurance that regurgitation in an infant is normal. Keeping the infant in a more upright position for 20 to 30 minutes after feeding (e.g., in an infant seat) will help control regurgitation.

PYLORIC STENOSIS

Pyloric stenosis affects approximately one male infant in every 150. It is considered to be more common in first-borns and four to five times more common in boys than girls. Onset is usually in the second to fourth week of life, but may be delayed up to the third month, depending on the severity of the stenosis. The pathophysiology of pyloric stenosis involves a thickening of the circular muscle of the pyloric sphincter, elongation of the pyloric region, and hypertrophy and hyperplasia of the stomach antrum. The exact cause for these changes is unknown.

History

The primary symptom is vomiting after feedings, soon becoming projectile in nature. Vomitus is not bilious, but may contain blood. Vomiting may be intermittent or after every feeding. Stools become small, infrequent, and constipated. The infant remains hungry, drinking eagerly, and will often take another feeding right after vomiting. Weight loss or lack of weight gain occurs.

Physical Examination

Lethargy, irritability, and various levels of dehydration with poor skin turgor and sunken eyes are present. Visible peristalsis from left to right may be seen. Palpation of the abdomen may reveal a firm, mobile, nontender, olive-sized mass to the right of the umbilicus and below the edge of the liver. The mass can be felt most easily immediately after the infant has vomited.

Diagnostic Tests

If the pyloric mass is not easily palpated, the diagnosis is made by an upper gastrointestinal series showing delayed gastric emptying and a narrow, elongated pyloric canal. Blood chemistries may show hypochloremia, hyperkalemia, and metabolic acidosis due to electrolyte losses from vomiting.

Management

Suspicion of pyloric stenosis needs to be referred for surgical evaluation and correction.

GASTROESOPHAGEAL REFLUX

Gastroesophageal reflux (GE reflux), repeated regurgitation of gastric contents into the esophagus, begins in the newborn period and is thought to be due, in part, to weakness of the esophageal sphincter. Hiatal hernia is frequently associated. The disease course is usually benign, with 60% of the cases resolving spontaneously by 6 months of age when the infant is more upright during the day and solid foods are introduced. It has been proposed that sudden infant death syndrome (SIDS) may be related to GE reflux, with death due to aspiration of refluxed material.

History

Recurrent vomiting or significant regurgitation after feeding is the most common sign. Vomiting may be forceful and possibly blood-tinged. Failure to thrive, dysphagia, irritability, pain, and colic may be present. Though uncommon, aspiration pneumonia may occur with complaints of night cough, wheezing, or apneic spells.

Physical Examination

Most signs and symptoms arise directly from the exposure of the esophageal tissue to the refluxed stomach contents. Depending on the severity of reflux and length of time before medical attention, the infant may be quite ill or fairly healthy. Anemia, hematemesis, and/or guaiac-positive stools all may be found. Irritability and abnormal posturing of the neck and torso (e.g., head tilt) may be the main reasons the infant was brought to the clinic.

Diagnostic Tests

In mild cases with a healthy infant, thorough history and physical examination are often sufficient for diagnosis. In other than mild cases, an upper gastrointestinal (GI) series is indicated. Esophageal pH testing and endoscopy are performed if upper GI study is inconclusive.

Management

Moderate to severe GI reflux warrants referral to a physician for confirmation and initial management. Postural elevation at a 45 to 60 degree angle is effective in 90% of cases, and is the main form of medical mangement. If reflux is severe, 24-hour-a-day positioning may be needed, but otherwise elevation of one to three hours after feeding is sufficient. Small, frequent, cereal thickened feedings (milkshake consistency) are given. Antacids between feedings are used if esophagitis is present.

Surgery is indicated only in cases of esophageal stricture, recurrent pneumonia, or severe pseudoneurologic symptoms, and in cases where adequate medical management has failed to achieve weight gain and control of emesis after six weeks of treatment.

DIARRHEA

Diarrhea is one of the most common complaints presented in a pediatric practice. Diarrhea itself may be the main problem or may be symptomatic of another underlying disease process. Diarrheal diseases continue to be one of the major causes of morbidity and mortality in children. When considering diarrhea, the nurse practitioner should be aware of the numerous diagnostic possibilities, yet not lose sight of the fact that the majority of diarrhea is benign and self-limiting. Infants and young children are particularly susceptible to more serious problems with diarrhea due to the low reserve capacity of their intestine and the fact that fluid and electrolyte losses may quickly lead to electrolyte imbalance, dehydration, and shock.

Since all causes of diarrhea need to be considered simultaneously, this topic will best be discussed in terms of acute infectious versus noninfectious diarrhea and the differing etiologies, workups, and management of each.

ACUTE INFECTIOUS DIARRHEA

As for most abdominal complaints, a detailed history is of prime importance in diarrhea. Information on frequency, duration, presence of blood or mucus, and color, consistency, and number of stools needs to be obtained. Vomiting, appetite, recent food or drug intake, similar symptoms in other family members, and the presence of fever or other symptoms are important items in the history.

A thorough physical examination is also required, with special attention directed towards looking for other infectious processes that may be causing diarrhea, (e.g., otitis media, pneumonia, and streptococcal pharyngitis). Examination of the stool for mucus, blood, or pus is important. Careful attention must be paid to the child's state of hydration, checking skin turgor, mucous membranes, fontanels, weight, and level of consciousness.

VIRAL GASTROENTERITIS

The majority of all diarrhea in North America is of viral origin. Rotavirus, adenovirus, ECHO virus, and Coxsackie virus are a few of the many viral agents causing gastroenteritis. Onset is acute and frequently accompanied by irritability, vomiting, crampy abdominal pain, and low-grade fever. Stools are loose but do not usually contain mucus or blood. Physical examination reveals hyperactive bowel sounds and mild diffuse abdominal tenderness. Symptoms resolve within three to four days with gradually diminishing diarrhea.

Management

Management consists of diet alteration and early supportive measures. If vomiting is present, all food and fluid intake is withheld for three to four hours; then clear liquids are introduced slowly and continued for 24 hours. In children, diet is advanced as tolerated to a bland or BRAT diet (bananas, rice cereal, applesauce, toast), then to a regular diet. An infant's diet, after 24 hours of clear liquids, may be advanced to half-strength formula, then to full strength as tolerated. Electrolyte rich fluids (Pedialyte, Gatoraid) are especially important in young children and infants. If dehydration is present, intravenous (IV) fluids are needed and the child should be referred appropriately.

Drugs are seldom needed and may in fact delay recovery if used excessively. Suspensions of kaolin (Kaopectate) or bismuth subsalicylate (Pepto-Bismol) may be used. Paregoric is not advised in younger children with vomiting due to the potential masking of surgical conditions. Diphenoxylate hydrochloride with atropine sulfate (Lomotil) has little place in the treatment of simple gastroenteritis.

BACTERIAL GASTROENTERITIS

Approximately 10% of infectious diarrhea is caused by a bacteria. *Salmonella, Shigella,* and strains of *E. coli* are enterovasive organisms and produce disease by penetrating the mucosa of the bowel. Enteropathogenic *E. coli* and *Staphylococcus* produce diarrheal disease by means of endotoxins. *Staphylococcus aureus* is seen in food poisoning and causes abrupt onset of vomiting, diarrhea, and prostration after two to six hours incubation period. Treatment for *S. aureus* food poisoning centers on maintaining fluid and electrolyte balance.

The other three organisms (*Salmonella, Shigella, E. coli*) are the main causes of bacterial infections. They produce similar symptoms and can only be positively identified with a stool culture. The incidence of bacterial enteritis is highest in children under 6 years old, and peaks between 6 months and 2 years. Infectious *Salmonella* organisms may be picked up from several environmental sources, most commonly from pet turtles, birds, or rodents, and from eating uncooked poultry, raw eggs, or spoiled mayonnaise. Transmission is by fecal-oral route from contaminated food and water. Incubation period is 12 to 24 hours. *Shigella* is endemic in the population with human carriers only. Transmission is also via the fecal-oral route. A history of travel or exposure may provide clues to *Shigella* infection.

The bacterial infections produce moderate to high fever, vomiting, watery diarrhea, malaise, abdominal cramps, and poor feeding. Stools often contain blood and mucus, with leukocytes present microscopically. Stools of *E. coli* are green and foul-smelling. White blood cell counts may be elevated with a shift to the left. Physical examination may reveal splenomegaly along with hyperactive bowel sounds and some diffuse abdominal tenderness. Diagnosis is made on the basis of stool cultures, and antibiotic therapy is best withheld until the specific pathogen has been identified.

Management

Management of *Shigella* and *Salmonella* infections is with ampicillin 100–150 mg/kg/day. Treatment of *Salmonella* infection is mainly done to prevent sepsis in the infant and the immunocompromised client but not to shorten the duration of the disease. Neomycin 100 mg/kg/day is used in *E.*

coli infections. Fluid and electrolyte balance must be watched carefully and be adequately maintained. Very ill or dehydrated children need referral for intravenous (IV) therapy and possible hospitalization.

NONINFECTIOUS DIARRHEA

Antibiotic Associated

In recent years, more postantibiotic diarrhea has been recognized. Any antibiotic may cause diarrhea and other GI problems, but the broad-spectrum antibiotics like the erythromycins, tetracyclines, ampicillins, and clindamycins are more frequently indicted. Associated GI symptoms are nausea, vomiting, bloating, cramping, and pruritis ani. Gastrointestinal symptoms usually begin about four days after antibiotic treatment was begun, but may begin as late as two weeks after antibiotic therapy was discontinued. Most patients respond well when antibiotics are withdrawn.

A rare although potentially dangerous side effect of antibiotic therapy is the development of colitis or pseudomembranous colitis. Severe diarrhea with blood, mucus, and pus; fever, leukocytosis, and possible dehydration and electrolyte imbalance characterize this condition. Immediate referral to a physician for careful treatment and follow-up is necessary since the disease may become life-threatening.

CHRONIC DIARRHEA

There are numerous disease processes and mechanisms that can cause chronic diarrhea (diarrhea lasting for more than two weeks) in children. Often the search is drawn out and puzzling, with numerous tests involved. The diagnosis and treatment of most chronic diarrheal diseases is not within the scope of the nurse practitioner, so these areas will only be briefly touched upon for the purpose of intelligent initial evaluation and referral.

As in any chief complaint of diarrhea, a thorough history of the disease is important (see acute infectious diarrhea). In chronic diarrhea, the growth and developmental status is particularly important. Normal growth and weight patterns are unlikely if the disease process is organic. It is important to conduct a thorough physical examination to look for other diseases that may cause chronic diarrhea, (e.g., diabetes and hyperthyroidism). It is necessary to make sure the child is indeed having diarrhea and not experiencing watery leakage around impacted stools.

The extent of the diagnostic tests naturally depends on what the history and physical examination reveals. A stool culture and examination usually is done first to look for bacterial infections, ova and parasites, fat particles, blood, stool pH, and reducing substances. Blood chemistries and a sweat chloride test are also appropriate. Endoscopy, upper and lower GI series, roentgenograms for bone age, and other miscellaneous blood, urine, feces, and pancreatic tests are performed as needed.

The differential diagnosis includes several broad etiologic categories of chronic diarrheal disorders. The major diseases within each category will be mentioned, accompanied by a brief overview of therapy.

Malabsorptive Diseases

Although the malabsorptive diseases represent a small percentage of diarrheal illness in children, they continue to be a major cause of disability and growth retardation. Cystic fibrosis, celiac disease, and the various deficiency diseases, (e.g., disaccharide deficiency), are included in this category. Steatorrhea, bulky, foul-smelling stools, failure to thrive, abdominal pain and distension are all symptoms of malabsorptive diseases. Most malabsorptive diseases involve a malfunction in the small bowel.

Cystic fibrosis has an incidence of about 1 in 1,500 and is the most common malabsorptive syndrome of infancy and childhood. The infant has a good appetite, but weight gain is poor. Multiple respiratory infections, a distended abdomen, wasted buttocks, and clubbed fingers may occur. The disease is diagnosed by a sweat test showing an excessive amount of sodium chloride. Treatment involves dietary and vitamin supplementation and pancreatic enzyme replacement.

Celiac disease (gluten-induced enteropathy) has an approximate incidence of 1 in 3,000, although estimates vary widely. The onset of symptoms is around 6 months of age when gluten is first added to the diet. Fat malabsorption results; the appetite is poor, abdomen distended, and buttocks wasted. Anemia and growth retardation frequently occur. Diagnosis is by small bowel biopsy. Treatment is a lifelong gluten-free diet (i.e., no wheat, rye, oats, or barley).

The sugar malabsorptive diseases (mono- and disaccharide deficiencies) are not uncommon in certain ethnic groups (e.g., Negroes, Asians, Eskimos, and American Indians). The primary symptom is watery diarrhea after consumption of the offending sugar. The malabsorption may be congenital or acquired, with the acquired syndromes often resolving after a few weeks. Acquired or secondary lactase deficiency is a more common malabsorptive disease and may occur after any disease that damages the small intestine, (e.g., gastroenteritis). Diagnosis is by sugar-loading tests and estimations of fecal sugar. Treatment is by eliminating the offending sugar from the diet.

Inflammatory Bowel Disease

Crohn's disease (regional enteritis) is an uncommon, chronic inflammatory disease of the bowel and is characterized by recurrent attacks of abdominal pain and diarrhea. Fever, anemia, weight loss, and growth retardation are generally present. Extraintestinal symptoms of arthritis, erythema nodosum, or stomatitis may occur. This disease has a higher incidence among Jewish people. The onset is generally in early adolescence. The physical examination may reveal tenderness and a mass in the right lower quadrant. Diagnosis is made by an upper GI series and barium enema. The disease course is progressive and marked by exacerbations and remissions throughout life. Treatment is best handled by a gastroenterologist and involves multifaceted therapy with diet control, drug therapy, steroids, and supportive physical and psychological care.

Chronic ulcerative colitis is an inflammatory bowel disease marked by diffuse inflammation and ulceration of the mucosa of the colon and rectum. The disease is characterized by recurrent attacks of bloody diarrhea, rectal bleeding, and crampy abdominal pain. As in Crohn's disease, fever, weight loss, growth retardation, and extraintestinal symptoms of arthritis, erythema nodosum, and stomatitis are commonly found. Physical examination reveals an ill, malnourished patient. The abdomen may be distended; rectal tenderness is present; large numbers of leukocytes are present in the stool. Differentiation between colitis and Crohn's disease is at times difficult, but colitis generally has bloody diarrhea and pain in the left lower quadrant, as opposed to the right lower quadrant tenderness and diarrhea without blood found in Crohn's disease. Diagnosis is made by sigmoidoscopy and barium enema. Treatment involves diet and drug therapy, supportive care, and steroid use. Surgery (total proctocolectomy) is curative and is considered if medical management has failed.

Irritable Colon Syndrome

Irritable colon syndrome, or chronic nonspecific diarrhea, is one of the most common causes of chronic diarrhea in a child. Typically, a healthy, thriving child of 6 to 20 months of age begins having several loose mucoid stools during the day. The child was usually a colicky infant and there may be a family history of functional bowel disorders. The diarrhea is not greatly affected by the diet except for intake of low residue foods. Periods of stress, infection, or excessive stimulation seem to worsen the symptoms.

Physical examination is normal, revealing a healthy growing child with a good appetite. Laboratory tests and stool examinations are normal. The diagnosis is generally made by excluding organic problems. Treatment is aimed at reassuring the parents that the condition is not organic or disabling and will usually resolve by 4 years of age. Elimination of iced foods and fluids and between-meal snacks may help lessen diarrhea symptoms.

Milk Allergy

The uncommon condition of cow's milk intolerance is more often found in boys and families with a history of allergies. Symptoms usually begin before

6 weeks of age and involve abdominal distension, fever, diarrhea, and edema. Atopic dermatitis, urticaria, and asthma may also occur. Stools contain obvious or occult blood. Anemia and failure to gain weight frequently occur. Laboratory tests are generally unhelpful. The diagnosis is supported with milk challenge tests. Elimination of cow's milk from the diet corrects symptoms. Milk allergy usually resolves spontaneously by 2 years of age, but care should be exercised whenever new foods are introduced.

CONSTIPATION

SIMPLE/INCIDENTAL CONSTIPATION

Constipation is a common occurrence in childhood and usually results from faulty dietary habits, disruption of the child's routine, or a painful anal fissure that causes stool withholding. Dietary habits include too little free water and inadequate intake of high residue foods. Large quantities of milk may be constipating due to the low residue and high calcium content. Events disrupting the child's normal defecating routine, such as long trips, social events, or simply the child's refusal to come in from play, result in stool holding, which can lead to constipation.

History and Physical Examination

The diagnosis is made by the physical examination and a history of hard or infrequent stools. Physical examination may reveal a slightly distended abdomen or palpable feces in the abdomen. Rectal examination reveals hard feces. Special care should be taken during the examination to rule out a fissure.

Management

Treatment is aimed at helping the child to pass the hard stool and preventing recurrence; this is done by diet alteration to soften the stool. Increasing intake of fresh fruits and vegetables, free water, and natural laxatives (e.g., prune juice, apricots, tomatoes) may be sufficient to soften the stool and correct the initial constipation as well as prevent its recurrence. Adding a teaspoon of dark Karo syrup to an infant's formula may also help. A glycerine or Dulcolax suppository or oral mineral oil (15 ml) may be used to help pass a hard stool. A Fleet enema or manual removal of impacted feces may be necessary. If anal fissures are present, the above measures should be instituted as well as sitz baths. Mineral oil or suppository use may be needed until the fissure is healed.

ACQUIRED MEGACOLON

Bowel emptying depends on a defecation reflex which is initiated when stool fills the rectum and stimulates the pressure receptors of the rectal muscle. Defects in filling or, more commonly, in emptying of the rectum causes constipation. As stool remains in the rectum, water is reabsorbed leaving the stools hard and the ampulla of the rectum stretched, thus requiring more filling of the rectum to stimulate pressure receptors. A vicious cycle of constipation, hard stools, and painful defecation leading to stool holding and further constipation may ensue, resulting in a condition of acquired megacolon. The defecation reflex in early childhood seems easily disrupted by something as minor as a long trip, or by a psychologically stressful event, such as toilet training or the birth of a sibling. At times, there is a constitutional predisposition to constipation that helps to initiate the cycle leading to megacolon. Whatever the original episode, a self-perpetuating cycle ensues, resulting in severe fecal retention, hard stools, and distended rectal muscles.

History and Physical Examination

A detailed history of infancy bowel habits and the onset of symptoms is important. Psychological or family stress may be present or may have occurred at the time of constipation onset. Chronic abdominal pain, poor appetite, and lethargy are common client/guardian complaints. Encopresis, in which watery fecal material leaks around impacted stool, may be confused with incontinence, diarrhea, or willful soiling. Abdominal distension or palpable feces may be present on examination. The rectum is full of hardened stool.

Management

The goal in treating acquired megacolon is to keep the rectum empty most of the time. This permits the enlarged ampulla to shrink to normal size, thereby allowing the musculature to tighten up and normal defecation to resume. Diet alteration to increase bulky fibrous foods and fluids is encouraged. Sufficient quantity of mineral oil (15 ml taken two to four times daily) to produce four to five stools a day should be given initially. The dose should then be reduced to twice daily to keep the feces soft and the bowel lubricated for easy passage of stool. This helps the child to learn that passing stool is not a painful process and to overcome willful stool withholding. Treatment with mineral oil should be continued for several months to establish regular bowel habits. A stool softener (Colace) should then be used as needed to prevent recurrence of constipation.

Establishing a regular bowel movement pattern is done by placing the child on the toilet for a period of time after meals (taking advantage of the gastrocolic reflex) or at regular intervals, whether or not anything results.

CONGENITAL MEGACOLON

Hirschsprung's disease is one of the most common causes of intestinal obstruction in the newborn period. More common in males, it results from a segment of bowel lacking parasympathetic ganglion cells. Peristalsis cannot occur in the aganglionic segment, leading to obstruction and failure to pass stool.

History and Physical Examination

Vomiting, abdominal distension, irritability, and anorexia in a newborn who has failed to pass meconium is the typical picture of Hirschsprung's. Vomiting may become bilious and then fecal. Stools are loose and infrequent. Breathing may be difficult due to severe abdominal distension. In some cases, symptoms may appear later and resemble those of partial obstruction. Diarrhea, obstipation or chronic constipation, and failure to thrive are common in the older child. On examination, the rectum is empty of stool.

Management

Suspicion of Hirschsprung's disease requires immediate referral. Treatment is surgical removal of the aganglionic segment with a colostomy/ileostomy. Later resection of the bowel is done in some cases.

PARASITES

There are many parasites that cause disease in humans. Most parasites are responsible for only minor discomforts to the client; however, if neglected, parasites can cause significant morbidity and even mortality. The pediatric population is more vulnerable to parasitic infections due to greater exposure to infected soil as well as the very young having no natural immunity to these invaders. With age, humoral and cellular resistance occur and the rates of morbidity and mortality drop significantly.

ENTEROBIASIS (PINWORMS)

Pinworms are one of the most common of the parasitic infections; it is estimated that nearly 20% of all children in the United States harbor the worm. Transmission is anal-oral, from direct contact, or from contaminated clothes or environment.

History and Physical Examination

Anal itching, especially at night, is the primary symptom of pinworms. The worms reside in the cecum and colon, with the females crawling out at night to deposit their eggs around the anus. The pinworms may also infect the vagina of females and result in vaginal discharge and itching.

Diagnostic Tests

Diagnosis is made by observing the ova or adult worm. Pressing a transparent (Scotch) tape around the anus in the morning and then examining it under the microscope may reveal eggs that the tape has picked up. Live worms or ova may be seen in the stool. A reliable parent can also be instructed to look between the buttocks with a flashlight after the child has been sleeping in the dark for one to two hours. An accurate description or collection of the worms warrants treatment.

Management

Pyrantel pamoate (Antiminth), mebendazole (Vermox), or piperazine citrate (Antepar) are all effective in eradicating the infection. Due to the high rate of cross-infection, treatment of the whole household is recommended. Frequent laundering of pajamas, linens, and undergarments in hot water is important. Nails should be kept short and clean and good handwashing techniques practiced.

ANCYLOSTOMIASIS (HOOKWORM)

The hookworm is generally found in tropical and temperate regions only. The eggs are excreted in feces and the larvae develop in the soil. A human may come in contact with the larvae by walking barefoot in or handling contaminated soil. The larvae penetrate the skin, migrate via the bloodstream to the lungs and up the pharynx, and are then swallowed. The larvae develop into adult worms in the intestine.

History and Physical Examination

Itching and a papular rash may be present where the larvae penetrated the skin. With heavy infections, abdominal pain, distension, and changes in the bowel habits may occur. In children, apathy, pallor, anorexia, and growth failure are also common. Since hookworms live off blood, an iron deficiency anemia may be present.

Diagnostic Tests

Diagnosis is made by finding the hookworm ova in the stool.

Management

Treatment is with pyrantel pamoate (Antiminth) or mebendazole (Vermox). Wearing shoes in endemic areas is advised.

ASCARIASIS (ROUNDWORM)

The roundworm ova are harbored in the soil after being passed in the feces. Ingestion of contaminated soil allows the ova to hatch into larvae in the intestine. The larvae then enter the bloodstream, circulate through the lungs, are coughed up and swallowed, and then return to the intestine to develop into adult worms.

History and Physical Examination

Due to the passage through the lungs, respiratory symptoms of asthma, cough, and upper respiratory infection may be produced. Weight loss, low-grade fever, abdominal pain, and anorexia may also occur. Eosinophilia may be present.

Diagnostic Tests

Diagnosis is made by a history of passing a large round worm in the stool or by presence of the ova in a fecal smear.

Management

Eradication of the worms is accomplished with pyrantel pamoate (Antiminth), mebendazole (Vermox), or piperazine compounds (Antepar); the disease, however, is usually self-limited to a year, even without treatment.

TRICHINOSIS

The larvae of *Trichinella spiralis* are found in the muscle of hogs and may be ingested by humans if pork is inadequately cooked.

History and Physical Examination

A history of abdominal pain, vomiting, and diarrhea within 48 hours after consuming poorly-cooked pork is the typical acute picture. Symptoms may be severe or mild. Chills, fever, weakness, a rash, edema of the face and eyes, splinter hemorrhages, and headache may occur. Splenomegaly upon examination is not uncommon. Muscle pain occurs when the migrating larvae enter muscle tissue and become encysted.

Diagnostic Tests

The characteristic triad of muscle pain, periorbital edema, and eosinophilia is sufficient to make a presumptive diagnosis of trichinosis. There are several serologic tests for trichinosis, as well as a skin test, that help support the diagnosis. Muscle biopsy showing encysted larvae is the most definitive test at the present time.

Management

Supportive measures are indicated since no specific treatment exists. Hospitalization and steroid use may be indicated for severe acute symptoms. Recent use of mebendazole (Vermox) has shown some promise in treating trichinosis infections. Thiabendazole (Mintezol) is also used with some success, although the side effects are numerous and the clinical response varies.

TAENIASIS (TAPEWORM)

Beef or pork *Taenia* larvae enter the human host when undercooked beef or pork is eaten. The larvae develop into adult tapeworms in the intestine where they then attach themselves via suckers to the gut mucosa. Larvae may also enter the bloodstream and circulate to the muscle tissue where they become encysted (cysticercosis).

History and Physical Examination

Symptoms are generally absent, with infection revealed only by tapeworm segments in the feces. Diarrhea, fever, abdominal pain, excessive appetite, and failure to gain weight may occur. Cysticercosis may be manifested only when subcutaneous or muscle nodules develop.

Diagnostic Tests

Diagnosis is made by seeing tapeworm segments in the stool, or by demonstrating ova in the fecal smears.

Management

Treatment is with niclosamide (Yomesan) or, as a second choice, quinacrine (Atabrine Hydrochloride), both of which are best followed by a saline enema.

GIARDIASIS

The protozoa *Giardia lamblia* is one of the most frequent causes of parasitic malabsorption in the United States. It is transmitted in food and water, or from person to person. Campers and hikers who drink from streams and those who travel abroad are more likely to be affected, although the pathogenicity is variable and poorly understood.

History and Physical Examination

Giardia infections may be asymptomatic or produce only mild gastrointestinal upset. Diarrhea, prolonged if untreated, is one of the primary symptoms of the disease. The stools may be bulky, greasy, and foul-smelling as gut malabsorption may occur. Symptoms of bloating, anorexia, vomiting, and abdominal pain may be present.

Diagnostic Tests

Diagnosis is made by identifying the *Giardia* trophozoite in fresh stool; however, in only 50% of the cases is the protozoa found. The diagnosis can also be made by using the string test (Enterotest) to obtain duodenal fluid for identification of the protozoan. If giardiasis is suspected, often a therapeutic trial of metronidazole (Flagyl) is used to clarify the picture.

Management

Metronidazole is the drug of choice with quinacrine hydrochloride as an alternative. Supportive measures to restore nutritional and fluid balance are used.

STUDY QUESTIONS

Circle all that apply.

Jeff S., a high-school senior, comes to your clinic this morning complaining of severe lower right side abdominal pain that began yesterday and has gotten steadily worse. Jeff limps in slowly, holding his side, and does not want to stretch out fully on the examination table. He appears pale and in a good deal of pain. The pain is much worse when he moves or takes a deep breath. He took some aspirin without relief. He vomited this AM, although he had not eaten anything. His last bowel movement was two days ago. Oral temperature is 100.4° F, pulse 94, respirations 26. You suspect an acute appendicitis.

1. What things in the history would suggest such a diagnosis?

     a. location of the pain
     b. pain quality and duration
     c. mild fever and vomiting
     d. general appearance and reluctance to move
     e. age

2. With further examination and laboratory studies you would expect to find:

     a. positive psoas sign
     b. mild leukocytosis (10–15,000 WBC/cu mm)
     c. abdominal flaccidity and guarding
     d. right-sided tenderness on rectal examination
     e. bluish discoloration of the lower right of the umbilicus

Bobbie L., a previously healthy 9-month-old boy, is brought to the afternoon clinic by his mother who says that Bobbie has been having "screaming fits" today and he can't be consoled. These "fits" began suddenly early this morning. He has had four "fits" which lasted 5 to 10 minutes. After the "fit" he seemed to be okay again, although tired. After this last screaming episode, though, he didn't look as good. Mrs. L. thinks he may have a stomachache since he didn't want to eat and "he kept his legs drawn up" for a while after the crying episode.

     On exam, Bobbie is pale, listless, and weak. His abdomen is slightly distended and a sausage-shaped mass is palpable in the right upper quadrant. Rectal temperature is 101° F. (Bloody stool was noted on the thermometer.)

3. Intussusception

     a. requires immediate referral for reduction
     b. is more common in girls
     c. is a common cause of obstruction in children less than 3 years old
     d. is characterized by recurrent attacks of abdominal pain, bloody bowel movements ("currant jelly stools"), and progressive weakness

4. Recurrent abdominal pain is characterized by all of the following except:

   a. is rare in the pediatric age group
   b. has a strong psychosomatic basis
   c. pain has no relationship to activity, eating, or bowel movements
   d. treatment is with mild anticholinergics and antispasmotics
   e. stressful events may precipitate or exacerbate the pain

   Ms. W., an 18-year-old mother, brings her first child, 2-month-old Sally, to the clinic because of frequent "vomiting" after eating. Sally has "done this since she was born."

5. What other information would you want to ask Ms. W. about Sally?

   a. type of food/formula eaten
   b. information on feeding techniques
   c. description of emesis (e.g., amount, timing, forcefulness)
   d. presence of other symptoms (e.g., pain, cough, irritability)

   Physical examination reveals a healthy, happy, growing infant. Sally takes a bottle so eagerly, according to Ms. W., that she doesn't even get a chance to burp Sally before the milk is all gone. Sally takes about 6 ounces of formula every four to five hours for a total of 32 ounces a day. Ms. W. has also been giving her some apple juice since "Sally likes it a lot." Stools are normal, without blood or mucus. Vomiting occurs directly after feeding when the child is being burped, or after Sally has been laid down. She vomits about 1 to 2 tablespoons of curdled milk at a time. Sally is in the 97th percentile on the weight curve and 70th percentile on the length curve.

6. Which of the following would you want to tell Ms. W.?

   a. infant regurgitation is normal up to 9 months of age
   b. Sally's problem involves normal regurgitation exacerbated by too much formula, eating too quickly, infrequent burping, and introduction of juices too early
   c. laying the child down on her stomach to allow her to rest after eating may decrease the spitting up
   d. an upper GI is needed to rule out other problems, (e.g., pyloric stenosis or GE reflux).
   e. burping Sally after every 1 to 2 ounces of formula taken may decrease regurgitation and slow down her eating rate
   f. switch Sally to whole milk since the heavier milk protein is not as easy to spit up

7. The primary symptom of pyloric stenosis is:

    a. small, tightly-formed stools
    b. excessive intake of fluids
    c. vomiting after feedings
    d. retention of body fluids
    e. bloody diarrhea

8. On palpation of the abdominal region, which of these findings are suggestive of pyloric stenosis?

    a. no pathologic signs
    b. nontender, moveable mass below the liver and to the right of the umbilicus
    c. soft, stationary mass to the right of the umbilicus
    d. abdominal tenderness in the right upper quadrant
    e. visable peristalsis from left to right

Jeff F., a 3-year-old boy was brought to the clinic by his mother because of a lack of bowel movements over the past five days. Before that, he experienced some pain on defecation. His mother reports that his last stools were small and tightly formed. Vital signs are normal.

9. In taking the history, which of the following would be important clues to the child's current complaints?

    a. history of past bowel habits
    b. presence of family/personal stress or differing activities
    c. eating habits
    d. sleeping habits
    e. appetite and activity level

Your physical examination reveals that the rectum is full of hardened stool and the abdomen is slightly distended. No fissures are seen. Jeff's mother also reports the client experienced a moderate stressor at the daycare center seven days ago.

10. Which is the most likely diagnosis?

    a. simple constipation
    b. acquired megacolon
    c. congenital megacolon
    d. Hirschsprung's disease

Six weeks later, Jeff returns because mother says his constipation has worsened after being treated the first time. Now he has bowel movements every 7 to 10 days and cries the whole time. They have had to use enemas at times "to get him to go at all." Stools are hard and dry. Bowel movements have become a real source of tension for the family and child. Physical examination is normal except for the rectum being full of hard and dry stool. You correctly suspect an acquired megacolon.

11. Which of the following are appropriate treatment measures?

    a. Fleet enemas qod to keep the rectum clean
    b. increase dietary intake of fresh fruits and vegetables
    c. increase intake of milk and dairy products
    d. mineral oil for several weeks to keep the stools soft and easily pass-
       able
    e. bowel retraining

12. Congenital megacolon (Hirschsprung's disease) is characterized by:

    a. failure to pass meconium
    b. bilious vomiting and abdominal distension
    c. hematuria and melena
    d. hypertrophy of ganglion cells in the colon
    e. rectum full of hard stool

    You are seeing 18-month-old Christy K. in your office for the chief com-
    plaint of diarrhea since yesterday with vomiting one time this morning.
    She remains active and playful although her appetite is down. She "felt
    warm" yesterday but her temperature was not taken.

13. What other information do you want to find out about Christy's illness?

    a. exposure to similar illness or similar symptoms in the family mem-
       bers
    b. description of the stool (e.g., blood or mucus in it)
    c. other symptoms (e.g., earache, sore throat)
    d. recent food or drug intake, especially antibiotic intake
    e. state of hydration

14. Which of the following would be signs of dehydration in Christy or a
    younger child?

    a. crying tears
    b. fontanels sunken in infancy
    c. excessive drooling
    d. decreased skin elasticity
    e. dry diaper for 12 hours

Christy's mother reports no other symptoms or intake of medicine or spoiled foods. Her 5-year-old brother had some loose bowel movements and stomachaches four days ago, but he is well now. No blood or mucus has been noted in the stool. Christy's physical examination is normal except for some slightly hyperactive bowel sounds. She is not dehydrated. Rectal temperature is 100° F. You decide to treat this as a viral gastroenteritis.

15. Which of the following, if found, would have made you suspect a gastroenteritis of bacterial origin instead of viral?

   a. normal temperature
   b. streaks of blood and mucus in the stool
   c. family owning several turtles and hamsters
   d. history of family traveling outside of the country
   e. WBCs in the stool

16. Christy's treatment consists of:

   a. clear liquids for 24 hours
   b. paregoric for the diarrhea
   c. advancement to a BRAT diet when tolerated
   d. stopping all dairy products and fried or spicy foods until well

   Five-year-old Randy L. is brought to the clinic by his mother because he has been scratching his buttocks for about two weeks. He says it itches a lot. Mother says she saw a small, moving worm that looked like a "skinny grain of rice" in his bowel movement this morning. Appetite and activity are unchanged. Physical examination is normal.

17. The type of parasite responsible for Randy's itching is most likely a:

   a. pinworm
   b. roundworm
   c. liver fluke
   d. trichinosis infection

18. Pinworm infection is characterized by which of the following?

   a. pruritis ani, especially at night
   b. diarrhea and stomach cramps
   c. pinworm eggs laid outside the body around the rectum
   d. rarely contagious
   e. ova may be visualized in fecal smears

15-year-old Kim Y. appears with the complaint of diarrhea for two weeks. She has also been feeling "bloated," although her appetite is poor and she has not felt like eating much. She says her stools are smelling worse and worse. No blood or mucus has been noted in them, however. Clear liquids and Kaopectate have not helped any. No abnormal food intake is recalled, except what she ate on a church backpacking trip three weeks ago. They hiked along a "real clean" river for four days, which is where they obtained their water. Symptoms began shortly after returning home. The physical examination is normal, although Kim has lost 2 pounds.

19. The history and physical examination suggest what type of disease?

    a. viral gastroenteritis
    b. bacterial gastroenteritis
    c. giardiasis
    d. food poisoning
    e. nematode infection

20. Which of the following is/are true of trichinosis infections?

    a. infection begins after eating poorly-cooked pork containing the *Trichinella* parasite
    b. the larvae may penetrate the muscle tissue and become encysted
    c. a triad of eosinophilia, muscle pain, and periorbital edema is typical symptomatology of trichinosis
    d. bloody diarrhea is a frequent symptom
    e. vomiting, diarrhea, and abdominal pain are common acute symptoms

ANSWERS

1. all	11. b, d, e
2. a, b, d	12. a, b
3. a, c, d	13. all of the above
4. a, d	14. b, d, e
5. a, b, c, d	15. b, c, d, e
6. a, b, e	16. a, c, d
7. c	17. a
8. b, e	18. a, c, e
9. a, b, c, e	19. c
10. a	20. a, b, c, e

BIBLIOGRAPHY

Conn, H. F., & Conn, R. B. (Eds.), *Current diagnosis*. Philadelphia: W. B. Saunders, 1977.

Davidson, M. GI problems in children, part I. *Hospital Practice,* August 1976, *47.*

Davison, P. F. GI problems in children, part II. *Hospital Practice,* September 1976, *105.*

Glouberman, S. Recurrent abdominal pain in children. *Arizona Medicine,* 1980, *37, 3,* 158–160.

Graef, J. W., & Cone, T. E. (Eds.). *Manual of pediatric therapeutics*. Boston: Little, Brown, 1974.

Kempe, C. H., Silver, H. K., & O'Brien, D. (Eds.). *Current pediatric diagnosis and treatment* (5th ed.). Los Altos, CA.: Lange Medical Publications.

Michener, W. M., Ament, M. E., & Hamilton, J. R. Gastrointestinal problems in children. *Audio-Digest Pediatrics,* 1980, *26,* 14.

Ramirez-Ronda, C. H. Antibiotic-associated colitis and diarrhea. *Forum on Infection,* 1976, *3,* 15.

Stickler, G. B., & Murphy, P. B. Recurrent abdominal pain. *American Journal of Diseases of Children,*1979, *133,* 486.

Vaughan, V. C., McKay, R. J., & Behrman, R. E. (Eds.). *Nelson's textbook of pediatrics* (11th ed.). Philadelphia: W. B. Saunders, 1979.

Walker, W. A., & Sondheimer, J. M. Advances in pediatric gastroenterology. *Audio-Digest Pediatrics,* 1978, *24, 3.*

CHAPTER 9

DIABETES

Anne L. Turner

Insulin-dependent diabetes mellitus (IDDM), formerly called juvenile-onset, ketosis-prone diabetes, is a chronic illness in which the onset is seen primarily in childhood. In 1975, the National Commission on Diabetes reported that approximately 5% of the U.S. population had diabetes, including both diagnosed and undiagnosed cases. Twenty percent of diabetes is the insulin-dependent type. A large proportion of insulin-dependent diabetes is seen with an onset in childhood.

Diabetes mellitus can be broadly defined as a condition manifested by an inappropriately high blood glucose level (hyperglycemia) due to either absolute insulin deficiency (decreased pancreatic beta cell insulin production) or decreased insulin effectiveness (increased peripheral resistance to insulin effects, circulating insulin antagonists), and associated with complications of microangiopathy, neuropathy, nephropathy, and macrovascular disease.

Diabetes can occur at any age during childhood, although it is rarely seen in infancy. There are two age periods, 5 to 6 years and 11 to 13 years, where a peak incidence of new cases can be expected (1). There is no sex preference. Diabetes is the most common serious endocrine problem in children. The etiology of IDDM is unknown but several studies have suggested a viral, immunologic, or genetic cause.

HISTORY AND PHYSICAL EXAMINATION

The onset of IDDM is rapid. Symptoms may include polyuria, polydipsia, rapid weight loss with unusual hunger, blurred vision, and fatigue. Parents

This work was supported by National Institutes of Health Grant No. P60 AM 20593.

may note the symptom of polyuria expressed as nocturia or as enuresis in a previously toilet-trained child. They may also recall symptoms of polyuria, polydipsia, and weight loss several weeks before the acute onset of diabetes in the child. Some clients may have diabetic ketoacidosis often associated with an intercurrent infection. The physical exam, in the absence of an acute illness, is essentially negative with the exception of marked weight loss and possibly dehydration, if mild to severe ketosis is present.

DIAGNOSTIC TESTS

Diagnosis of IDDM in children is based on the presence of the classic symptoms of diabetes (i.e., polyuria, polydipsia, rapid weight loss) together with a random blood glucose greater than 200. Laboratory data at diagnosis should include elevated blood glucose, positive urine ketones and glucose, or electrolyte imbalance, if ketoacidosis is present. The standard oral glucose tolerance test is rarely necessary for the diagnosis of diabetes in children (2).

MANAGEMENT

Hospitalization of the child is usually necessary at the time of diagnosis of diabetes. Goals of hospitalization include: to normalize blood glucoses and restore metabolic balance; to establish an insulin dose regimen; to develop a diet plan; and to provide education and emotional support for the child and parents.

Treatment of IDDM always includes insulin as well as diet and exercise. The treatment goals for each child should be individualized and include the following:

1. Metabolic control with plasma glucose levels as close to normal as possible
2. Maintenance of normal growth and development
3. Promoting the child's full participation in self-care activities appropriate to the child's age
4. Structuring the treatment regimen to allow the client to live as productive a life as possible
5. Reducing the risks for long-term complications

The amount of participation by the pediatric nurse practitioner in the care of the child with diabetes is dependent on the institution. In many cases, the pediatric nurse practitioner will be mainly responsible for education and counseling, whereas in other institutions the nurse practitioner may be the primary care provider. The means of attaining the goals, as described above, are described in the following sections.

COUNSELING

A chronic disease such as diabetes, cannot be treated with drugs alone but requires a regimen of diet, medication, and exercise. Success in adhering to this regimen requires the client to have a basic understanding of the illness and its treatment. The nurse practitioner in the clinical practice can easily integrate the client's medical management along with the education of diabetes self-care. Client education is an essential and vital part of the treatment plan.

The daily management of diabetes must be handled by the client; therefore, it is essential that he or she possess certain self-care skills. There are several skills that are essential for the diabetic to attain in order to minimally manage on a day-to-day basis. These can be referred to as survival skills, basically technical skills, which include the following:

1. Mixing and administering appropriate dose of insulin
2. Home monitoring of urine/blood glucose and urine ketones; knows when to contact the health care provider for abnormal test results
3. Knowledge of symptoms and treatment of hypoglycemia
4. Knowledge and ability to adhere to a basic diet plan
5. Knowledge of sick day rules and symptoms of uncontrolled diabetes
6. Knowledge of foot care

The educational process for the child with diabetes should always include the parents, as well as other significant family members (e.g., siblings, grandparent living at home with the child). The child should be encouraged to accept responsibilities for self-care as determined by the child's age and level of maturity. The young school-age child (6 to 8 years old) can generally perform urine tests with parental supervision, and the older school-age child (9 to 10 years old) should be encouraged to give the insulin injections. Encouraging the child to take responsibility for certain self-care skills promotes independence and will lessen dependence on parents during the teenage years.

The teenage years present special problems with diabetes. The teenager strives to develop an identity and acceptance among his/her peers. The label of "diabetic" can cause feelings of isolation, denial, and rejection in the teen. During teen years, the youth may try to cope with these feelings by ignoring the diabetes. Problems with diabetic self-care noncompliance are especially prevalent during the teen years. In counseling the teenager, the pediatric nurse practitioner should try to provide reasonable alternatives to the diabetic regimen (e.g., urine tests with the dipstick method rather than the two drop copper reduction method, or changing to blood glucose testing). The teenager should be encouraged to interact with other teens with diabetes to support positive peer identity.

Other areas that should be included in the educational program for the child with diabetes are long-term management of metabolic control (e.g., how to change insulin doses when appropriate), knowledge of possible long-term complications; and, knowledge of community resources for the child with diabetes (e.g., diabetes summer camps, American Diabetes Association, Juvenile Diabetes Association, support groups). In many communities there are diabetes education programs to which the nurse practitioner may refer the clients. The reader is referred to the end of the chapter for a listing of client education resources.

PHARMACOLOGY

INSULIN

Clients with IDDM are dependent on daily injected insulin to prevent ketosis and preserve life. There are various forms of insulin available and the most commonly used insulins are listed in Table 9.1. Insulin is available in concentrations of U40 (40 units per 1 cc volume) and U100 (100 units per 1 cc volume) with the latter the most commonly used.

For most clients, beef and pork insulin is the conventional type. Pure pork and pure beef insulins are available for those with allergies. Pure pork insulin often is used to treat lipodystrophy, which is seen more commonly in children and young women. Lipoatrophy is a complication of insulin therapy used in cases where there is a loss of fat tissue at the injection site and sometimes at other sites where insulin has not been administered.

Table 9.1. Commonly Used Insulins

Name	Type	Onset of Action	Peak	Duration
Regular	Short-acting	1/2–1 h	2–3 h	5–7 h
Semilente	Short-acting	1/2–1 h	4–7 h	8–10 h
NPH	Intermediate	2–4 h	8–12 h	18–24 h
Lente	Intermediate	2–4 h	8–12 h	18–24 h
Ultralente	Prolonged	4–8 h	16–18 h	36 h
Protamine zinc (PZI)	Prolonged	4–8 h	14–20 h	36 h

Abbreviations: NPH, neutral protein Hagedorn.

Hypertrophy, an accumulation of adipose tissue at the injection site, is often due to repeated injections at one site. Avoidance of the hypertrophied area by rotation of injection sites, the primary treatment, should be encouraged, and pure pork insulin may be necessary (3).

The main goal in insulin therapy is to normalize blood glucose levels (both minimizing hyperglycemia and avoiding frequent hypoglycemia), and there are several treatment regimens used to accomplish this goal. The regimen selected should be tailored to meet the client's metabolic needs as well as life-style. Institutions of insulin therapy should only be done with the consultation of a physician.

Most authorities agree that the child with diabetes can be managed best on at least one to two injections per day in a combination of short-acting (Regular—Lente) and an intermediate-acting (NPH—Lente) insulin. The generally accepted ratio for the total daily dose split into two injections per day is morning dose of 2/3 to 3/4 and an evening dose of 1/3 to 1/4 (of the total daily dose). The ratio of short-acting insulin to intermediate-acting insulin in the morning dose is usually 2/3 to 3/4 intermediate-acting; 1/3 to 1/4 short-acting insulin. The evening dose is generally divided into 1:1 ratio mixture of short-acting to intermediate-acting insulin.

At diagnosis, the child may require from 0.5 to 3.0 units/kg body weight/ day, depending on the severity of metabolic imbalance (4). Insulin requirements usually fall rapidly after diagnosis once the metabolic status is stabilized. During the remission (honeymoon) phase, the child may require less than 0.5 units/kg/day as endogenous insulin production continues. The length of the remission phase can vary from a few weeks to several months. Constant glucose monitoring and adherence to the diet plan is essential during the remission phase, since endogenous insulin production may decline abruptly. After the remission period, insulin requirements will climb steadily to 0.5 to 0.7 units/kg/day (4).

Adjusting insulin doses in the child should be based on home blood/urine glucose records, weight and height growth, patient's report of hypoglycemia/

Table 9.2.   Guidelines in Adjusting Insulin Dosage

Time of Occurrence	Hyperglycemia	Hypoglycemia
AM	* ↑ PM intermediate	† ↓ PM intermediate
12 N	↑ AM short-acting	↓ AM short-acting
PM	↑ AM intermediate	↓ AM intermediate
HS	↑ PM short-acting	↓ PM short-acting

* ↑ = increase dose or add that type of insulin
† ↓ = decrease that type of insulin dose

hyperglycemia symptoms, diet, and exercise patterns. The nurse practitioner may use the following as general guidelines for adjusting insulin doses:

1. Look at patterns of glucose control (daily home urine/blood glucose records)
2. Adjust only one insulin (type) at a time
3. Wait four to five days before making another adjustment
4. Change the dose by no more than approximately 10% of the total daily dose

The reader is referred to Table 9.2 for a description of adjusting specific insulins according to hypoglycemia/hyperglycemia patterns.

Consider the following client situations as examples in adjusting insulin doses:

EXAMPLE 1. Seven-year-old girl with IDDM for two years. Morning dose is 8 units NPH, 2 units Regular insulin. Evening dose is 4 units Regular insulin. Dose/kg/day is 0.55. Height and weight appropriate for age. Urine glucose records are as follows:

AM	12 N (%)	PM	HS
Neg	3	1/2%	Neg
Trace	5	1%	1/2
Trace	5	1/2%	Trace
1/2%	3	Trace	Neg

The 12 noon urine sugars are high, which indicates inadequate coverage by the morning dose of short-acting insulin (Regular). The total dose of insulin appears to be adequate based on the child's weight. The dose should be changed by adding 2 units Regular to the morning dose, bringing the total morning dose to 8 units NPH, 4 units Regular).

EXAMPLE 2. Thirteen-year-old with IDDM for one year. Morning dose is 14 units NPH, 8 units Regular insulin and an evening dose of 8 units Regular insulin. Total dose is 0.6 units/kg/day. Diet is adequate for normal growth and development. Urine tests are as follows:

AM	12 N	PM (%)	HS
1/2%	—	5	1%
Trace	Neg	3	1/2%
Trace	Neg	5	Trace
Neg	—	3	1%
1/2%	—	5	1%

Insulin dose is appropriate for age and weight, but urine test records indicate afternoon hyperglycemia. As a child enters adolescence, insulin dose requirements may increase up to 1.0 unit/kg/day. In the absence of afternoon hypoglycemia symptoms, the morning dose should be increased to 16 units NPH, 8 units Regular insulin.

EXAMPLE 3. Sixteen-year-old with IDDM for eleven years. Morning dose is 20 units NPH, 14 units Regular insulin, and evening dose is 10 units Regular insulin. Total dose is 0.85 units/kg/day. Client is compliant with diet and complains of nocturia. Blood sugar results as follows:

AM	12 N	PM	HS
300	—	100	160
240	80	120	—
400	200	180	240
400	—	120	200

Complaints of nocturia along with morning hyperglycemia indicate inadequate coverage from the evening insulin dose. Adding NPH insulin to the evening dose will provide better night coverage. The evening dose should be changed to 4 units NPH, 10 units Regular insulin.

EXAMPLE 4. Morning dose is 10 units NPH, 4 units Regular insulin and the evening dose is 4 units NPH, 4 units Regular insulin. Height and weight appropriate for age.

AM	12 N (%)	PM (%)	HS
Neg	Neg	Neg	Neg
5%	—	1/2%	Trace
5%	—	1/2%	Neg
5%	Neg	Neg	Neg
5%	—	Trace	Trace

Client complains of nightmares and early morning headaches.

This example of urine sugar results represents the somogyi (rebound) effect. The client's complaints of early morning headaches and nightmares indicate nocturnal hypoglycemia. As the blood sugar level falls during the night, hormones (adrenalin, glucagon, growth hormone, and cortisone) stimulate gluconeogenesis, thus producing a high blood sugar level. Urine test results would indicate heavy glucosuria alternating with negative urine sugars and sometimes nonspecific complaints of hypoglycemia. The evening dose should be changed to 2 units NPH, 4 units Regular insulin.

DIET

Diet is an important variable in the treatment plan for the child with diabetes if normal growth and development are to be maintained along with metabolic control. A dietitian (R.D.) should always be consulted to aid in designing an appropriate diet plan and to provide long-term follow-up for necessary changes in the diet plan. There are three important factors in the diet plan for the child with diabetes: (*1*) a consistent caloric and nutrient daily intake (e.g., kcal, carbohydrate, protein, fat); (*2*) a nutritionally balanced diet with strict avoidance of concentrated sweets (e.g., candy, regular soft drinks, Jello, sugar); and (*3*) proper distribution of meals throughout the day—three meals and two to three snacks.

The dietary plan should be tailored to meet the child's growth and development needs as well as individual preferences. The parents should be instructed that the daily caloric intake must be consistent and meals or snacks should never be delayed (eaten within one hour as prescribed) or skipped. This may pose special problems for the adolescent, for example, who may refuse to eat a midmorning snack during the school term. Every effort should be made to tailor this plan for the client's individual preferences.

Special occasions, such as sick days, eating out, holidays, and extra exercise should also be areas included in the diet plan. The parents should be instructed on special meal plans for sick days (e.g., substituting liquid sugar foods for the usual diet when ill) (5). Several references are available for children/parents about eating out (e.g., fast food restaurant exchange lists) in the American Diabetes Association publication, *Diabetes Forecast*. Holiday meals (e.g., birthdays, Thanksgiving) present special problems and individual discretion should be used. Extra or strenous exercise requires extra calories (carbohydrates) before the exercise. A dietician (R.D.) should be consulted to aid the child and family in planning for these special occasions.

MONITORING CONTROL

The criteria for acceptable diabetic control are still very controversial, although most agree now that maintaining blood glucose at a near normal range can reduce the risks of long-term microvascular complications (6). Diabetes control in the child with IDDM is assessed by laboratory measures, client's report of hypoglycemia/hyperglycemia symptoms, the child's growth and development (specifically height and weight), and the client's daily home monitoring of glucose control.

Laboratory measures used to monitor diabetes control include blood glucose, urine glucose, and glycosylated hemoglobin (HbA_1). The type of laboratory measure used by the PNP in the ambulatory care setting is dependent on the institutional preference. Blood glucose may be measured as either fasting or postprandial levels. Some authorities aim for fasting levels less than 120 mg% and two hour postprandial glucose levels less than 150 mg%. Goals for blood glucose levels should be individualized for each child, but a general goal is to get the blood glucose as close to normal as possible. Measuring urine sugars in the IDDM client should not be used as the primary tool for assessing control. The average renal threshold for spilling glucose ranges between 150 to 180, although these values can vary significantly in individuals. High renal thresholds are more commonly seen in the elderly; lower renal thresholds, although rare, can be seen in the young child (i.e., child spills glucose in the urine when blood glucoses are less than 150 mg%). Measuring a blood glucose along with a second voided urine glucose may aid in determining an estimate of the client's renal threshold.

Glycosylated hemoglobin (HbA_1), a relatively new laboratory measure, provides an important tool in assessing diabetic control. The assay measures the amount of glucose bound to the hemoglobin molecule during the red blood cell's 120-day life-span. The test provides an objective measure of glucose control for a period of four to six weeks and is an important tool, particularly for the insulin-dependent client whose blood glucoses may be subject to wide fluctuations. The nurse practitoner should consult the clinical laboratory for normal values since these are dependent upon the type of assay used. Goals for glycosylated hemoglobin levels for the IDDM client should be individualized with the general goal of striving for near-normal values.

The child's height and weight also glucose should be monitored as a measure of diabetes control. Standard growth charts that plot height and weight on the basis of age and percentiles should be used. Uncontrolled diabetes may be exhibited by the child not following the standard growth curves for weight or height. Also abnormal weight gains could signify excessive insulin dosages. Deviations in height growth should be discussed with the physician as these may signify poorly controlled diabetes or other endocrine problems.

The client's home monitoring of daily glucose control is an extremely important variable in assessing diabetes control. The child with IDDM should be instructed to check either urine or blood glucose levels two to four times daily. The client monitoring urine glucose should use the two-drop copper reduction method (Clinitest) which measures urine sugars up to 5%. Home blood glucose should be monitored in the client whose renal threshold is variable or high, who is experiencing difficulty with control, who is non-compliant with urine testing, or the client who wishes to do blood monitoring at home. Home blood glucose monitoring can also be used to supplement urine glucose testing and to detect hypoglycemia or when the urine glucoses are high. Home blood glucose monitoring can easily be accomplished using either strips (Chemstrip bG, Visidex) or with a meter (Statek or Glucometer). Urine ketones should be monitored when the blood/urine sugar is high or when the client is ill. It is essential that the client keep written records and the nurse practitioner should review these with the client at each visit.

In summary, insulin-dependent diabetes mellitus is a chronic illness in which the onset is rapid and most commonly seen in childhood. The condition is due to a decreased or absolute lack of insulin production. Some children may present in diabetic ketoacidosis, or the diagnosis may be made after the parents note hyperglycemia symptoms. Clients with IDDM are dependent on daily injected insulin to prevent ketosis and to preserve life. The prescribed diet plan should be designed to promote normal growth and development, along with maintaining metabolic control and meeting individual preferences. Monitoring diabetes control includes laboratory measures, client's report of hypoglycemia/hyperglycemia symptoms, the client's growth and development, and the client's daily monitoring of glucose control. Acute and chronic complications of IDDM and client education will be discussed in the later section of this chapter.

COMPLICATIONS

Most authorities agree that a relationship exists between good versus poor metabolic control and the development of long-term complications. While one major aim in diabetes management is to keep the client symptom free, controversy still exists in determining criteria for describing control. Good control (defined as maintaining euglycemia) appears to decrease the incidence of refractive changes, prevent certain types of infection, promote normal growth and development in children, and possibly reduce congenital defects in the newborn of the pregnant diabetic woman (7).

It is still uncertain if good control will prevent the complications due to microangiopathy, although evidence is growing to support the concept that reduction of blood glucose levels can decrease the risks for microvascular complications (6). Some have suggested that genetic factors, insulin, or some other abnormality in metabolism other than hyperglycemia is responsible for the development of complications (7). Maintaining good metabolic control is essential along with routine screening to guard against the development of complications. Although the development of long-term complications due to diabetes (retinopathy, nephropathy, neuropathy) is not commonly seen in the young, the pediatric nurse practitioner should be aware of the clinical manifestations and include screening as a routine part of the treatment plan. This section will discuss acute and chronic complications of diabetes.

ACUTE COMPLICATIONS

Acute complications of diabetes generally are due to hypoglycemic coma, diabetic ketoacidosis, or infection. The child and family should be instructed in the symptoms, treatment, and prevention of hypoglycemia. Additionally, the parents should be instructed in the use of glucagon for the treatment of severe hypoglycemia.

Minor acute illnesses, such as colds or the flu, can present difficult problems for the insulin-dependent client. The child and family should be instructed in the management of the diabetes on sick days. Illnesses create an added stress and hyperglycemia may result. (Refer to *An Instructional Aid*

Table 9.3.   Sick Day Management*

Everyone gets sick now and then. Sometimes tooth problems, a cold, or the flu can present special problems in managing your diabetes. Below are guidelines that can help you manage your diabetes on sick days.

1. Always take your insulin. You may even need to take extra doses of Regular insulin (short-acting). Consult your health care provider for instructions on taking extra insulin doses.

2. Check your urine/blood for glucose and urine for ketones at least every four to six hours and keep a record of the results. Notify your health care provider if your urine glucose stays high or if you have continuous amounts of moderate to large ketones in the urine.

3. Drink plenty of liquids (especially calorie-free, sugar-free drinks). Liquids are usually well-tolerated during sickness and prevent dehydration. Try to drink at least 6 to 8 ounces every hour.

4. Call your health care provider immediately if you start vomiting, have persistent diarrhea, or if the illness does not improve after 48 hours.

5. If you do not feel like eating your regular-size meal, eat smaller amounts of food more often. Soft, easy-to-chew, or liquid foods are tolerated well.

6. When you have nausea or diarrhea, it may be necessary to replace the regular diet with liquids. For insulin-dependent diabetics, this will mean drinking liquids with some sugar in them. Examples of suitable liquids are fruit juice, gingerale, or regular cola. Regular Jello, popsicles, ice cream, and soup also may be eaten. It is usually best to take these in small amounts (e.g., $1/4$ to $1/2$ cup) as frequently as can be tolerated.

*Christensen, N. K. and Turner, A. L., *Patient Instructions for Sick Day Management.*

on Juvenile Diabetes, for a further discussion of sick-day management) (5). Table 9.3 lists instructions for clients and families to aid them in the management of minor acute illnesses at home.

Diabetics are more prone to infections. Infections commonly seen in the child with diabetes include vaginal candida infections, urinary tract infections, and occasionally, skin infections in the form of boils. Screening for infections should be a part of each visit.

CHRONIC COMPLICATIONS

Retinopathy

Diabetic retinopathy is the leading cause of new blindness in the 20 to 64 age group. The prevalence of retinopathy is positively correlated with the duration of diabetes (i.e., the longer the duration of diabetes, the higher the prevalence of retinopathy).

Retinopathy can be described as a weakening of blood vessels on the retina and is usually divided into two stages: nonproliferative and proliferative retinopathy. Nonproliferative (or background) retinopathy is characterized by intraretinal and retinal vascular permeability changes (8). Ophthalmoscopically visible signs of background retinopathy include microaneurysms, exudates, and cotton wool spots. The client may not note any visual changes if the macula is not involved. The second stage, proliferative retinopathy, is characterized by the growth of new retinal blood vessels which are weaker vessels. It is thought that these vessels develop as a response to underlying retinal ischemia (8). The new vessels (neovascularization) are prone to bleeding, thus resulting in hemorrhages that cause visual disturbances (e.g., blindness can result if the hemorrhage is large). Treatment of proliferative retinopathy has shown great advancements in recent years with the development of photocoagulation (laser).

Surveillance is the most important issue for the pediatric nurse practitioner in caring for the child with diabetes. Retinal examinations using the ophthalmoscope offer only a limited view of the retina and are inadequate for routine screening for diabetic retinopathy. Stereoscopic fundus photographs offer larger views of the fundus and thus better surveillance. If fundus photographs are not available, the child should be referred to an ophthalmologist for retinal screening.

Nephropathy

Diabetic nephropathy is a serious and life-threatening microvascular complication of diabetes. This complication usually is seen after 10 to 15 years duration of diabetes and is usually asymptomatic until renal failure or nephrotic syndrome develops.

The nurse practitioner should routinely screen for diabetic nephropathy in all diabetic clients. The urine should be tested for protein (dipstick) at each clinic visit and a serum creatinine should be determined if the urine protein is positive. Immediate physician referral is essential for abnormal creatinine levels and persistent proteinuria. Additionally, the nurse practitioner should routinely screen for urinary tract infections. This may be accomplished by using a urine dipstick for nitrites. Positive urinary nitrites should always be thoroughly investigated with a urine culture and all urinary tract infections should be treated promptly. Chronic urinary tract infections will necessitate further urological workup.

Neuropathy

Diabetic neuropathy is a polymorphous group of syndromes which affect the nervous system. These syndromes may have an acute onset with a short duration or an insidious onset that is progressive to a chronic nature. The etiology of a neuropathy is unknown, but it is characterized by destruction of peripheral nerve axons and myelin damage, metabolic aberrations in the nerve, and abnormalities in nerve conduction. There is a wide range of manifestations which generally fall into four categories: distal symmetrical poly-neuropathy, autonomic neuropathy, proximal motor neuropathy, and cranial mononeuropathy.

The pediatric nurse practitioner may rarely see neuropathy manifested in his or her pediatric diabetic population. Distal symmetrical polyneuropathy is sometimes seen in the pediatric diabetic client after several years duration of the disease or during episodes of poorly controlled diabetes.

The client usually will first note pain and paresthesias. The client may complain of tingling, burning, aching, or pain in the feet occurring most often at night. Physical examination may reveal decreased perception of light touch, pain, vibration, and temperature in the lower extremities. Deep tendon reflexes may also be diminished in the lower extremities.

Improvement in peripheral neuropathy can be seen with improvement in the diabetes control. At the present time, there are no good medical therapies for the treatment of neuropathy, although some practitioners use carbamazepine, diphenylhydantoin, tricyclic antidepressants, or fluphenazine (Prolixin) for the treatment of pain due to neuropathy. The nurse practitioner should consult the physician before initiating drug therapy for neuropathy. Instruction in foot care, and especially in the prevention and care of foot wounds, is important for the client experiencing decreased sensation in the feet due to neuropathy.

CLIENT EDUCATION RESOURCES

AMERICAN DIABETES ASSOCIATION

The American Diabetes Association is a lay and professional organization concerned with client and professional education, research, and public awareness. Most communities have local chapters which offer various client services (e.g., educational classes, support groups) and have educational materials available. The national organization publishes a bimonthly journal, *Diabetes Forecast* which contains excellent articles for the client/family on diabetes care, diet, and new research findings.

JUVENILE DIABETES FOUNDATION

The Juvenile Diabetes Foundation is a lay organization primarily concerned with fund-raising for research. Some communities may have local chapters. The national office has printed educational materials for the insulin-dependent diabetic and parents.

NATIONAL DIABETES INFORMATION CLEARINGHOUSE

The Clearinghouse is a federally-funded organization which serves to collect, organize, and disseminate information about diabetes programs and educational materials.

STUDY QUESTIONS

Circle all that apply.

1. A parent brings her 5-year-old daughter to your office with complaints of enuresis. The child was toilet trained at the age of 3. What other symptoms might also indicate diabetes?

   a. polyuria
   b. weight gain of 6 pounds in two months
   c. polydipsia
   d. leg cramps
   e. vigorous appetite
   f. weight loss

2. A 16-year-old girl with IDDM for six years complains of pitting areas on her upper arms, abdomen, and thighs. She gives all her insulin injections in her thighs. The pitting areas are due to:

   a. hypertrophy
   b. allergy to metal needles
   c. poor site rotation
   d. lipoatrophy

3. John, a 13-year-old diabetic, complains of early morning headaches. His morning insulin dose is 16 units NPH, 10 units Regular and evening dose is 6 units NPH, 4 units Regular. His usual test results are AM: negative or 5%; supper: negative to 1/2%; and HS: negative to trace. What dose change recommendation would you make?

   a. change the morning dose to 14 units NPH, 10 units Regular
   b. change the evening dose to 4 units NPH, 4 units Regular
   c. change the evening dose to 8 units NPH, 4 units Regular
   d. change the evening dose to 8 units NPH, 6 units Regular

4. Distal symmetrical polyneuropathy is characterized by

a. absent deep tendon reflexes
b. facial twitching
c. pain and paresthesias in the legs
d. frequent hypoglycemia
e. decreased vibratory sense in the legs
f. pain in the legs, especially at night

Nedra, a 7-year-old with IDDM for one year, comes to your office for a routine visit. Her height and weight are appropriate for her age. Her morning insulin dose is 6 units NPH, 4 units Regular and evening dose is 2 units Regular. Her urine test records are as follows:

AM	12 N	PM	HS (%)
trace	neg	1%	3
1/2%	neg	1/2%	3
neg	—	neg	5
1/2%	—	neg	3
neg	—	1/2%	5

5. What would be the most appropriate dose change to make?

a. change the evening dose to 2 units NPH, 2 units Regular
b. change the evening dose to 4 units Regular
c. discontinue the evening dose
d. change the morning dose to 8 units NPH, 4 units Regular

ANSWERS

1. a, c, f
2. d
3. b

4. a, c, e, f
5. b

REFERENCES

1. Drash, A. L. The child with diabetes, in Rifkin, H. & Raskin, P. (Eds.) *Diabetes Mellitus, Volume V.* Bowie, Md.: Brady, 1981.
2. National Diabetes Data Group. Classification and diagnosis of diabetes and other categories of glucose intolerance. *Diabetes,* (1979), *28,* 1039–1057.

3. Galloway, J. A., & Davidson, J. D. Clinical use of insulin, in Rifkin, H. and Raskin, P. (Eds.) *Diabetes Mellitus, Volume V.* Bowie, Md.: Brady, 1981.

4. Drash, A. L. Diabetes Mellitus, in Vaughan, V. C. and McKay, R. J. (Eds.) *Nelson's Textbook of Pediatrics* (10th ed.). Philadelphia: W. B. Saunders, 1975.

5. Travis, L. B. *An Instructional Aid on Juvenile Diabetes Mellitus.* (6th ed.). Galveston, Texas: The University of Texas Medical Branch, 1980.

6. American Diabetes Association. Blood glucose control in diabetes. *Diabetes,* 1976, *25,* 237–239.

7. Rifkin, H., & Ross, H. Control of diabetes and long-term complications, in Rifkin, H. and Raskin, P. (Eds.) *Diabetes Mellitus, Volume V.* Bowie, Md: Brady, 1981.

8. Henkind, P., & Walsh, J. B. diabetic retinopathy, in Rifkin, H. and Raskin, P. (Eds.) *Diabetes Mellitus, Volume V.* Bowie, Md.: Brady, 1981.

BIBLIOGRAPHY

American Diabetes Association. Blood glucose control in diabetes. *Diabetes,* 1976, *25,* 237–239.

Christensen, N. K., & Turner, A. L. *Patient instructions for sick day management.* Vanderbilt Diabetes Research and Training Center, 1982.

Drash, A. L. Diabetes mellitus, in Vaughan, V. C. and McKay, R. J. (Eds.) *Nelson's textbook of pediatrics.* (10th Ed.). Philadelphia: W. B. Saunders, 1975.

Drash, A. L. The child with diabetes, in Rifkin, H., and Raskin, P. (Eds.) *Diabetes Mellitus, Volume V.* Bowie, Md.: Brady, 1981.

Galloway, J. A., & Davison, J. D. Clinical use of insulin, in Rifkin, H., and Raskin, P. (Eds.) *Diabetes Mellitus, Volume V.* Bowie, Md.: Brady, 1981.

Henkind, P., & Walsh, J. B. Diabetic retinopathy, in Rifkin, H., and Raskin, P. (Eds.) *Diabetes Mellitus, Volume V.* Bowie, Md.: Brady, 1981.

National Diabetes Data Group. Classification and diagnosis of diabetes and other categories of glucose intolerance. *Diabetes,* 1979, *28,*1039–1057.

Rifkin, H., & Ross, H. Control of diabetes and long-term complications, in Rifkin, H., and Raskin, P. (Eds.) *Diabetes Mellitus, Volume V.* Bowie, Md.: Brady, 1981.

Travis, L. B. *An instructional aid on juvenile diabetes mellitus.* (6th ed.). Galveston, Texas: The University of Texas Medical Branch, 1980.

CHAPTER 10

ANEMIA

Pamela K. Busher

Anemia is a condition in which there is a reduction in the circulating red blood cell (RBC) mass. The clinical definition is expressed in terms of concentration of hemoglobin (Hgb) or as a packed red cell volume (hematocrit [Hct]). A 10% decrease below the following norms would be considered an anemic state (1).

Age	HgB (gm/100 ml)	Hct (%)
1 month	16	53
3 months	11.5	38
6 months to 1 year	12	40
2 to 6 years	13	43
7 to 12 years	14	46

The pathophysiologic process of anemia can be conceptualized either as an excessive loss of RBCs, an inadequate production of RBCs, or an increased destruction of RBCs. The reticulocyte count, a hematologic lab test usually available to the nurse practitioner will aid in differentiating whether the problem arises from poor production or rapid loss. Reticulocytes, precursors of the mature erythrocyte (RBC), are released into the blood stream from the bone marrow and should make up approximately 1% of circulating RBCs. In the 3- to 6-month age group, however, the count may normally be as high as 3%.

RBC indices are a help to further classifying the process. The mean corpuscular volume (MCV) and the mean corpuscular hemoglobin (MCH) classify the size and the hemoglobin content of the RBC, respectively. Norms for children from newborn to 15 years of age are (2): MCV = 77–106; MCH = 25–38. Anemia can occur as an acute process or as a chronic condition. As such, the clinical picture will vary. The age of the patient, the presence of concurrent health problems, and the etiology, duration, and severity of the anemia will influence the clinical presentation.

IRON DEFICIENCY

Iron deficiency is the most common cause of anemia in children and is highest between the ages of 9 to 24 months. The etiology of iron deficiency anemia can be divided into four major categories: (1) deficient intake, (2) increased demand; (3) blood loss; and (4) impaired absorption.

HISTORY AND PHYSICAL EXAMINATION

All infants are at high risk for a deficient state in that their iron stores are adequate to last for only four to six months after birth. Recommended requirements to maintain a normal hemoglobin range are from 1 to 2 mg/kg/ day. The history should question for use of an iron fortified formula or a medicinal supplement. Cow's milk is a poor source of iron. In children, diet deficiency is the main cause of a low iron state.

The child's birth history is important in that low birth weight infants have an increased demand for iron. In addition to low iron stores, these children exhibit a rapid growth phase, without a supplemented diet, leading to anemia by 9 months of age. Prenatal factors, such as placental bleeding and twin-to-twin transfusions, can lead to blood loss and eventual anemia. Blood loss also can result from hookworms, gastrointestinal bleeding secondary to cow's milk hypersensitivity, and GI bleeding as a result of gastric mucosal changes occurring from iron deficiency itself.

Impaired absorption can result from malabsorption syndromes or chronic diarrhea. Food tolerance, stool quality and quantity, and familial history of such diseases should be reviewed.

Other high risk groups are menstruating females and adolescents on restricted diets or low calorie regimens. The history in female clients should screen for unusually heavy menstrual bleeding. The frequency and duration of the cycle, as well as the number of pads or tampons used per cycle, should be assessed in an attempt to quantify flow. A diet history should question the intake of iron-rich foods, including red meat, turkey, liver, and dark leafy vegetables. General symptoms that can be uncovered from the history include anorexia, listlessness, and irritability.

Physical signs will be few if the anemia is chronic and will be somewhat nonspecific even with moderate to severe anemia. Pallor is an important clue. Tachycardia, a blowing systolic murmur, and splenomegaly may occur with Hgb levels below 5 gm and/or a Hct of less than 25%.

DIAGNOSTIC TESTS

- *Complete Blood Count (CBC)*. This will reveal an Hct and Hgb below normal levels.
- *Reticulocyte Count*. The count is normal or minimally elevated.
- *RBC Indices*. The MCV and MCH values will be less than normal, showing a microcytic hypochromic anemia.
- *Serum Iron*. The normal value is 120μg/100 ml. In an iron deficient state, it will be less than 50 μg/100 ml.
- *Total Iron Binding Capacity*. The normal value is 250 μg/100 ml. In iron deficiency it will be greater than 450 μg/100 ml.
- *Percent Saturation*. The normal value is 20 to 55%. A value of less than 15% will occur in iron deficiency anemia.
- *Peripheral Blood Smears*. The RBCs will be hypochromic and microcytic.

MANAGEMENT

The iron deficient state is treated with medicinal ferrous sulfate preparations which are inexpensive. The usual dose is 5 to 6 mg/kg/day, given in three divided doses and continued for one month after normal values are achieved. Different preparations have varying contents of elemental iron and the dose should be calculated accordingly. Parenteral iron should be considered for clients who have compliance difficulties, poor oral iron tolerance, or malabsorption states.

The client and family member responsible for the administration of the medication should be instructed to administer the preparation with juice or milk to minimize irritation of the gastrointestinal tract. Any dietary factors contributing to the original deficiency should be corrected by careful dietary counseling, focusing on sources of iron. The child's intake of milk should be restricted after one year (especially if the source is cow's milk) to 1 pint per day.

If the iron deficient state is not corrected after adequate treatment of if a new deficiency develops soon after treatment, the client should be referred for a work-up to rule out any hidden bleeding or iron metabolism disorders.

Counseling of clients should center around prevention. Screening for high risk clients, such as low birth weight children and menstruating adolescents is appropriate. Use of iron fortified formula or iron supplementation during the first 12 months of life is essential for all children.

Consultation or referral should be obtained for clients with hematocrits of less than 25%, for clients less than 10 months of age, for a history of blood loss, for a family history of anemia due to other causes, for an abnormal RBC morphology, and for an abnormal physical examination not explainable by iron deficiency.

SECONDARY CAUSES

Myriad causes other than iron deficiency can explain anemia in the pediatric client. These will be less commonly encountered by the nurse practitioner and require referral to and management by an appropriate medical specialist. The nurse practitioner, however, must be able to screen for these conditions. For classification purposes, these secondary causes of anemia will be divided into the categories of (*1*) decreased RBC production, (*2*) increased RBC destruction, and (*3*) blood loss.

DECREASED RBC PRODUCTION

In the following conditions, the bone marrow is unable to produce an adequate number of RBCs to maintain the normal circulating volume. As a result, low reticulocyte counts will be found.

Megaloblastic Anemias

Megaloblastic anemias are usually a result of folic acid or vitamin B_{12} deficiency. The RBC indices will be increased. A decreased serum folate level or decreased serum B_{12} level will differentiate the two conditions. Folate deficiency is most common and can be caused by an inadequate diet, by decreased absorption, or by drug-induced inhibition of metabolism. The peak incidence is between 4 and 7 months of age. Vitamin B_{12} must combine with an intrinsic factor, a glycoprotein secreted by the gastric fundus, for absorption. The most common cause for a B_{12} deficient state is the lack of secretion of this factor, a condition known as juvenile pernicious anemia. Its peak incidence is between 9 months and 4 years of age. Other less common causes of the deficiency are destruction or inhibition of the B_{12}-intrinsic factor complex, receptor site abnormalities in the ileum, and inadequate intake.

Megaloblastic anemia management revolves around correction of the specific underlying defect, if possible. Diet deficiencies must be eliminated and patient follow-up is essential.

When folate deficiency is suspected, the history should question for adequate intake. Infants who are premature or who receive most of their nourishment from goat's milk or powdered milk are at high risk. Since certain drugs can inhibit absorption (e.g., phenytoin, phenobarbital), medication use should also be questioned. Symptoms of this deficiency include irritability, failure to thrive, chronic diarrhea, and thrombocytopenic hemorrhages in advanced cases. Signs and symptoms of vitamin B_{12} deficiency may include anorexia, irritability, listlessness, and a red, smooth, painful tongue. Neurologic effects, such as ataxia, paresthesias, hyporeflexia, Babinski responses, and clonus may be elicited from history and physical exam.

Thalassemia

Thalassemia anemias are a group of inherited disorders of hemoglobin synthesis, specifically, the globin chains. The resultant red cell is highly fragile and as such is susceptible to oxidation, both factors contributing to the hemolytic feature of this anemia. The thalassemias can involve any combination of chain synthesis defect and can be further grouped according to the heterozygous state (thalassemia minor) and the homozygous states (thalassemia major and thalassemia intermedia). They occur as microcytic hypochromic anemias and can be differentiated from iron deficiency by the presence of normal serum iron values and an abnormal peripheral smear. Transfusion therapy, chelation therapy to prevent iron overload, and splenectomy will comprise the treatment plan after referral to the appropriate physician.

In screening for thalassemias, a family history is essential. Thalassemia minor usually presents no symptoms, although splenomegaly may be present. Thalassemia major may appear with hepatosplenomegaly, lymphadenopathy, and enlarged tonsils and adenoids.

Aplastic and Hypoplastic Anemias

Aplastic and hypoplastic anemias appear with a spectrum of laboratory findings, depending on the condition and its severity. Aplastic processes generally will be accompanied by a pancytopenia. Pure red cell aplasia appears clinically with a normocytic normochromic anemia and a normal WBC and differential. Bone marrow studies are indicated for definitive diagnosis.

Aplastic anemia can be caused by drugs capable of bone marrow suppression, such as benzene derivatives and chloramphenicol. Other causes are radiation and infection, especially viral hepatitis (3). Red cell aplasia occurs early in infancy and may be either congenital or acquired. The congenital form, the Blackfan-Diamond syndrome, occurs in the first year of life and is treated with transfusions and corticosteroids. The acquired form usually requires no therapy, although transfusions may be necessary if the anemia is severe.

Pure red cell aplasia may have a genetic basis, so a family history may be helpful. Pallor is prominent in pure red cell aplasia as well as in aplastic anemia. Symptoms of pancytopenia in the latter condition, such as petechiae, multiple ecchymotic areas, and a decreased resistance to infection are clues.

Anemias of Renal Failure, Chronic Inflammation, and Chronic Infection

These three types appear as normocytic normochromic anemias. The etiology stems from the inhibition of bone marrow activity as a result of systemic disease, although the exact pathophysiologic mechanism is unclear. Abnormal laboratory findings specific to the underlying disease will assist in diagnosing these disorders. Again, the nurse practitioner's role is one of referral since treatment will consist of correcting the disease condition. Endocrine conditions and neoplasms can underlie anemia states as well and will be screened for in a comprehensive medical workup.

INCREASED RBC DESTRUCTION

The underlying problem in this group of conditions, known as hemolytic anemias, is a shortened RBC survival time. In response to a decreased life-span of erythrocytes, bone marrow activity increases and the reticulocyte count will exceed 2%. Normoblastosis also will be characteristic.

Anemias Due to Intrinsic Abnormalities of the Red Cell

Hereditary spherocytosis is associated with splenomegaly and RBCs that are spherical in shape. Differential diagnosis includes other congenital hemolytic states and will involve an elaborate family history. Laboratory tests, including a peripheral blood smear and osmotic fragility studies, will be necessary for a conclusive diagnosis. The nurse practitioner will refer any suspect client to a physician for such diagnostic tests and for treatment, which usually involves a splenectomy.

Glucose 6-phosphate dehydrogenase deficiency (G-6-PD deficiency) is a disease involving an enzymatic defect of the RBC resulting in eventual hemolysis. Diagnosis is made from demonstration of reduced G-6-PD cellular activity and treatment is largely preventive, that is, avoidance of hemolytic precipitants, and supportive, such as blood transfusions.

Sickle cell anemia is a disease characterized by an abnormal hemoglobin synthesis, which deforms the RBC by rendering it rigid. As such, the red cells obstruct small blood vessels thus causing the pain of infarction—the acute sickling crises. A new theory is that there is something sticky about the RBCs that makes them adhere to each other and obstruct the vessels. The presence of the abnormal hemoglobin can be identified by a sickle cell preparation in which RBCs are deoxygenated and exposed to reducing agents. This does not distinguish between the acute disease and the trait, so a more precise electrophoretic examination of the hemoglobin is required for definitive diagnosis. The peripheral smear will show the characteristic sickle-shaped RBC.

A family history regarding the presence of the trait or actual disease of sickle cell anemia is key in the history-taking. Otherwise the symptoms will appear as crises of thrombosis or sequestration. The presentation of thrombotic crises will depend on the site of infarct—abdominal pain, bone tenderness, swollen joints, monoplegia or hemiplegia, or polyuria should raise suspicion. Shock can occur due to a decreased blood volume in spleen sequestration crises. This disease occurs almost exclusively in the black population with 10% carrying the trait and 1% having the actual disease.

Anemias Due to Extrinsic Abnormalities Causing RBC Destruction

Destruction of intrinsically normal red cells can occur as a result of immunologic factors or mechanical injury. In the autoimmune hemolytic anemias, the client develops antibodies to his or her own red cells—antibodies found either on the RBC itself or in the serum. A Coombs test is required to detect antibodies in the suspect client.

Cell fragmentation as a result of mechanical injury can arise from numerous pathologic processes. Burns can result in spherocytosis as well as hemolysis. Prosthetic heart valves and rough endothelial surfaces in blood vessels as well as the heart can cause anemias characterized by a variety of abnormally shaped RBCs (4).

BLOOD LOSS ANEMIA

Much of the anemia due to chronic blood loss will result in an iron deficient state due to a decrease in hemoglobin iron stores. As such, the underlying blood and the iron deficient state should be treated. Acute blood loss will result in a clinical picture of a normocytic normochromic anemia with a reticulocytosis. More vigorous therapy is required, so immediate referral by the nurse practitioner is in order.

The anemia of blood loss can be screened for by taking a careful history for urinary tract bleeding (e.g., dark or red-colored urine), severe or chronic bouts of epistaxis, gastrointestinal bleeding (e.g., coffee-ground emesis, dizziness, dark-colored stools), or recent trauma. Physical signs, such as pallor, systolic murmurs, postural hypotension, positive stool guaiacs, and positive urine tests for blood should be sought.

DIAGNOSTIC TESTS

- *CBC* will identify the anemia with the presence of a low Hgb and/or Hct. A concurrent pancytopenia would be an indication of primary bone marrow disease. An elevated WBC would implicate a systemic infection as a possible etiology.
- *Reticulocyte count* will determine if the process is one of decreased marrow production (low reticulocyte count) or increased RBC loss (high reticulocyte count).
- *RBC indices* will classify the size and hemoglobin content of the cell.
- *Peripheral smear* is necessary to determine the morphology of the RBC.
- *Serum iron, total iron binding capacity, percent saturation* values will help to rule out an etiology of iron deficiency.
- *Serum B_{12} level,* if less than 100 pg per ml is diagnostic for B_{12} deficiency.
- *Shilling's test,* a 24-hour urine, is another diagnostic test for vitamin B_{12} or folic acid deficiency. It tests the patient's ability to absorb B_{12}. A normal value is 7% or greater. If the results show poor absorption, there is B_{12} deficiency. Normal results in the face of a macrocytic anemia indicate folic acid deficiency.
- *Coombs tests* detect antibodies in the patient suspected of having an acquired hemolytic anemia. The direct Coombs tests for the presence of the antibody on the patient's own RBC; the indirect Coombs tests for the antibody in the patient's serum.
- *Sickle prep* is a simple screening test to determine the presence of abnormal hemoglobin; it does not distinguish between the trait and the actual disease.

MANAGEMENT

The nurse practitioner's role in the secondary causes of anemia is one of a referral agent. Health maintenance of these patients, however, is within his or her realm. The following are specific points of management to be considered in the ambulatory setting:

Folate Deficiency

1. The usual treatment will consist of oral folic acid of 0.5 to 1.0 mg daily.
2. Patient education is essential regarding dietary sources of folate which include liver, spinach, lettuces, cabbage, and avocados, to name a few. Poor sources include beef, cow's milk, potatoes, and chicken.
3. Follow-up visits to monitor the client's status are important in management. The usual treatment period is for three to four weeks, but can last up to several months.

Vitamin B$_{12}$ Deficiency (pernicious anemia)

1. Prophylactic B$_{12}$ should be given to high risk clients, that is, those who have had gastrectomies or ileal resections (4).
2. Usual maintenance therapy consists of monthly intramuscular injections of B$_{12}$ of 200 to 100 μg (8).
3. Treatment is usually a lifetime program and should be emphasized to the client and family.

Thalassemia

1. In beta thalassemia minor, folic acid supplementation often maximizes RBC production and should be considered.
2. Iron replacement is not indicated. Such therapy may lead to an overload of iron stores.
3. These clients are at risk postsplenectomy for massive infections. All should receive Pneumovax routinely, except for children under 2 years of age. With the primary health care provider's approval, all clients should be on daily oral penicillin prophylaxis at a dose of 250 mg/day (4).
4. Cardiac abnormalities may develop in clients who have been overloaded with iron. Digitalis and diuretics may be necessary to maximize cardiac output. Antiarrhythmics, such as quinidine may be necessary to suppress chronic dysrhythmias (4).

Spherocytosis

1. In the event that the client requires a splenectomy early in life, immunization with Pneumovax will be necessary.

G-6-PD Deficiency

1. Avoidance of drugs that may produce hemolysis is a necessity. Examples of these drugs include a number of sulfa drugs, nitrofurantoin, phenacetin, probenecid, and several antimalarials (4).

2. Ingestion of the fava bean (broad bean) may cause intravascular hemolysis in some G-6-PD deficient people. This variant occurs between the ages of 1 and 5 years, most often in boys of Mediterranean or black descent. Avoidance of the bean is indicated.

Sickle Cell Disease

1. No specific treatment exists to prevent sickling of the susceptible cells.
2. Supportive care is the mainstay of treatment and includes prompt treatment of infections and preventive measures, such as routine Pneumovax immunization. The child with sickle cell disease who appears with a high fever should be hospitalized. Sepsis and meningitis are frequent complications and can progress to death within a short time. Pneumonia is the most common infection and requires IV antibiotics. Urinary tract infections and osteomyelitis occur in a significant number of afflicted clients. Prophylactic penicillin will be provided at the discretion of the health care provider. All of these children should be put on penicillin 250 mg bid the day before any dental or surgical procedure, the day of, and for three days following (4).
3. The nurse practitioner should be aware of cholelithiasis, aseptic necrosis of the head of the femur, retinal disease, and cerebral vascular accidents as possible complications. He or she should be alert for painful hips or shoulders, abdominal pain, visual disturbances, and neurologic defects.
4. Client's legs should be observed for ulcers on the medial or lateral aspect of the ankle. These can arise as a result of trauma or spontaneously. Referral to a medical specialist is appropriate. Treatment consists of wound culture, debridement, and appropriate antibiotic therapy. Zinc therapy and direct oxygen therapy may be required in addition to transfusions to promote healing.
5. All of these children should be screened for G-6-PD deficiency.
6. Folic acid therapy (1 mg/day) may be given as early as 6 months of age for an excessively low Hgb (less than 9 gm) and a severe reticulocytosis (4).
7. Maintaining an adequate fluid intake is important in these children since they are susceptible to hypovolemia.
8. Sickling crises—attacks of localized pain accompanied by fever—should be referred immediately to a hospital for further evaluation.
9. Health maintenance check-ups should include an evaluation of growth and development, a Hgb/Hct screen, and a reticulocyte count. The child can be seen as frequently as every month by the nurse practitioner for the first year and progress to an every other month schedule by the second year. Depending on the stability of the client, a schedule of every three to six weeks can be decided thereafter.

10. Client and family education is the most essential part of the practitioner's therapeutic regimen. The practitioner is in an appropriate position to provide ongoing support to all involved. The nature of the disease and its genetic implications should be discussed with an open nondirective attitude. The need for the frequent follow-up checks should be stressed and the child's progress emphasized. Symptoms that warrant immediate medical attention should be discussed. These include fever, cough, increasing pallor seen best in the mucous membranes, the development of jaundice in the sclera, or any change in behavior. The institution of physical limits are not necessary as the child will set his or her own. Above all, the child should be treated as a normal-functioning family member and not receive preferential or limiting restrictions.

Hemolytic Anemias (autoimmune)

1. Corticosteroids are the mainstay of therapy in syndromes characterized by IgG antibodies activated at 37°C (4).
2. Syndromes characterized by IgM antibodies that are activated at temperatures of 4°C are responsive to a warm environment. Avoiding cold weather and wearing warm clothing can minimize hemolysis.

Mechanical RBC Injury

1. Iron therapy at 5 mg/kg/day may be required to balance an ongoing hemolytic process.

STUDY QUESTIONS

Circle all that apply.

1. A young black mother brings her 1-year-old child into your clinic for a well-baby check-up. The mother is on a limited income. The child, an active, alert boy, is gaining weight on a diet of soft table foods, including potatoes, fruits, and a few vegetables and meats. The child drinks approximately 2½ pints of whole cow's milk per day. He receives no supplemental vitamins. The screening Hgb shows a value of 10 gm/100 ml. Physical exam and review of the systems is unremarkable. The most likely cause of this anemia is:

   a. iron deficiency
   b. chronic blood loss secondary to cow's milk ingestion
   c. sickle cell disease

2. Your plan would include (choose all that apply):

   a. sickle prep
   b. stool guaiac
   c. decrease the child's milk intake
   d. client education regarding iron-rich foods
   e. medicinal iron supplementation
   f. serum iron studies
   g. recheck Hgb in one month

3. Match the following types of anemias with the appropriate description:

   (1) thalassemia   a. microcytic, hypochromic
   (2) iron deficiency   b. normocytic, normocyromic
   (3) aplastic anemia   c. macrocytic
   (4) B$_{12}$ deficiency
   (5) acute blood loss

4. Which of the following foods have the highest value of iron?

   a. milk, turkey, eggs, liver
   b. beef, spinach, dried fruits and nuts
   c. fish, spinach, fresh fruits

5. A 13-year-old black boy enters your clinic complaining of a two-month history of malaise associated with bouts of dizziness, abdominal pains, constipation, and dark stools. He denies swollen glands, fever, chills, muscle weakness, ataxia, visual disturbances, or any recent exposure to infections. Physical exam reveals normal neurologic status, negative abdominal findings, and a harsh systolic murmur over the aortic area. Appropriate *initial* screening lab tests might include:

   a. Hgb/Hct
   b. WBC with differential
   c. RBC indices
   d. reticulocyte count
   e. stool guaiac
   f. sickle prep

ANSWERS

1. a   (4)-c
2. a, b, c, d, e, g   (5)-b
3. (1)-a   4. b
   (2)-a   5. a, b
   (3)-b

REFERENCES

1. Headings, D. *The Harriet Lane handbook: a manual for pediatric house officers*. 7th ed. Chicago: Year Book Medical Publishers, 1975.
2. Wallach, J. *Interpretation of diagnostic tests*. 3rd ed. Boston: Little, Brown, 1978.
3. Beck, W. *Hematology*. 2nd ed. Cambridge, MA: The M.I.T. Press, 1977.
4. Gellis, S., & Kagan, B. *Current pediatric therapy*. 9th ed. Philadelphia: W. B. Saunders, 1980.

BIBLIOGRAPHY

Beck, W., *Hematology*. 2nd ed. Cambridge, MA: The M.I.T. Press, 1977.

Davidson, S., Passmore, R., Brock, J., & Truswell, S. *Human nutrition and dietetics*. 7th ed. New York: Churchill Livingstone, 1979.

Gellis, S., & Kagan, B. *Current pediatric therapy*. 9th ed. Philadelphia: W. B. Saunders, 1980.

Headings, D., *The Harriet Lane handbook: a manual for pediatric house officers*. 7th ed. Chicago: Year Book Medical Publishers, 1975.

Hoole, A., Greenberg, R., & Pickard, C. *Patient care guidelines for family nurse practitioners*. Boston: Little, Brown and Company, 1976.

Nelson, W., Vaughan, V., McKay, J., & Behrman, R. *Textbook of pediatrics*. 11th ed. Philadelphia: W. B. Saunders Company, 1979.

Rakel, R., & Conn, H. *Family practice*. Philadelphia: W. B. Saunders, 1978.

Robbins, A., & Tamkin, J. *Manual of ambulatory medicine*. Philadelphia: W. B. Saunders, 1979.

Sheldon, S., *Pediatric differential diagnosis: a problem-oriented approach*. New York: Raven Press, 1979.

Wallach, J., *Interpretation of diagnostic tests*. 3rd ed. Boston: Little, Brown, 1978.

CHAPTER 11

URINARY TRACT INFECTIONS

Donna M. Behler

Urinary tract infections (UTIs) are common in childhood, second only to respiratory infections. They represent a range of clinical conditions all secondary to the microbial invasion of tissues from the urethral meatus to the renal cortex. The urethra (urethritis) and bladder (cystitis) comprise the lower urinary tract; the kidneys (pyelonephritis) are the upper urinary tract.

Symptomatic bacteriuria is associated with symptomatic infection of any structure(s) of the urinary system; asymptomatic bacteriuria is the colonization of the urine with bacteria. Approximately 80% of the infections are due to *Escherichia coli*. Most arise by the ascending route, entering via the urethral meatus with the turbulence of flow carrying organisms to the bladder. Upon the closure of the urethra, contaminated urine may be returned to the bladder. The bacteria may clear on its own within 48 to 72 hours or colonize in the area, for example, the urethra or bladder. The UTI is usually self-limited whether symptomatic or asymptomatic.

If there is decreased competence of the ureterovesical valve, the organisms enter the ureter ascending to the medulla and cortex and result in acute pyelonephritis. Recurrent infections may predispose the child to progressive renal damage with chronic pyelonephritis. Chronic pyelonephritis, however, is not usually the result of repeated UTIs.

The nurse practitioner will most commonly see uncomplicated infections, that is, no underlying structural or neurologic lesions. In the complicated infections, there are residual inflammatory changes requiring surgical intervention, for example, obstruction, stones, or neurologic lesions. In these infections, *E. coli* is replaced by other species, such as *Proteus*.

SYMPTOMATIC UTI

The incidence of symptomatic bacteriuria is highly age-related. At particular risk are the newborn, preschool girls, pregnant women, and women with diabetes mellitus.

NEONATES AND INFANTS

The newborn and infancy periods are the most significant in that UTIs may quickly lead to scarring and atrophy. UTIs in infants, especially boys, are common presentations of urinary tract anatomic problems, for example, urethral strictures and posterior urethral valves. The overall frequency is about 1%. This is the only time when the incidence is higher in boys —4:1.

PRESCHOOL

Symptomatic UTIs are relatively common in the preschool child, that is, about 1.5%, with the girls being infected 10 to 20 times more than boys. This is a crucial period since there is a high frequency of major urologic abnormalities among those with significant bacteriuria ($\geqslant 10^5$ organisms per ml of urine). Boys usually have more advanced renal disease by the time their illness is detected.

SCHOOL AGE

Children in the first three grades are more frequently infected. Over 5 to 6% of girls will have one or more episodes of significant bacteriuria. This incidence is about 1.2% with a 30:1 ratio of girls to boys.

The frequency of symptomatic UTIs is less than asymptomatic bacteriuria (ABU) at each age. Approximately 50% of children with ABU are estimated to have had previous UTIs, the majority being girls.

History

A thorough history is essential as children do not have classic UTI symptoms such as are found in adults. A history of previous UTIs, poor health, chronic disease, and medication use needs to be ascertained. As with the incidence, the symptoms exhibited are also age-related.

- Neonates and infants. The caregivers of the newborn and infant may report vomiting and diarrhea, fever, frequent damp diapers, trouble starting flow, weak stream, dribbling, failure-to-thrive (FTT), colic, and/or irritability.
- Preschool. The preschool child may have symptoms of fever, dysuria, hematuria, FTT, enuresis, abdominal pain, constipation, and/or pinworms.
- School age. The older child may have fever, dysuria, abdominal discomfort, flank pain, frequency, foul smelling urine, and/or sudden enuresis.

Physical Examination

A complete physical examination should be done, especially in the infant/child with nonspecific symptoms. As the child may have fever alone, other sources of infection must be sought, for example, otitis media.

The abdomen should be examined for tenderness, masses, suprapubic pain. Costovertebral angle percussion tenderness should be identified. The genitalia should be inspected for external irritation and discharge (may also be seen with vulvovaginitis, foreign body, pinworms).

Diagnostic Tests

The proper collection of a urine specimen is crucial. The nurse practitioner will want to inspect a urine sample that most adequately reflects the true condition of the urine in the bladder.

In infants, a clean-catch specimen is very unreliable as the false-positive rate of a single specimen may be as high as 25%. From ages 1 month to 3 years, suprapubic aspiration is the most appropriate. In the circumcised boy, cleaning the genitalia and getting a bagged urine specimen may be sufficient. After the age of 3, a clean-catch midstream urine should be obtained in a sterile container. By discarding the first few ml, there is less risk of contamination with *Staphylococcus, Streptococcus,* and diphteroids which may be normal flora in children.

Written instructions or drawings given to the caregiver are helpful if he or she will be obtaining the specimen. The urethral meatus and the surrounding area should be cleansed with liquid soap and rinsed with water-soaked sponges. In the uncircumcised boy, the foreskin should be retracted.

The first morning specimen is ideal, but often unrealistic. The specimen should be examined and cultured within one hour. If the specimen is left out over two hours, bacterial counts in a contaminated specimen may increase, the pH can be altered, and WBCs may decrease.

A urinalysis (macroscopic examination) and a microscopic examination of the urine are indicated. The greatest yield will be with the microscopic examination.

Urinalysis. Urinalysis is helpful in detecting renal or metabolic disease, is quick and inexpensive. General characteristics to observe include color, odor, and turbidity. The pH, blood, ketones, glucose, bilirubin, and protein can be obtained by dipstick interpretation.

1. *Color* is affected by the concentration of food, dyes, blood. The normal color is from clear yellow to amber. The following are alterations with possible causes:

Milky: pus cells, phosphate crystals, large all-vegetable meal
Dark yellow: concentrated urine
Nearly colorless: decreased normal urochrome pigments; may be forcing fluids
Yellow-brown to green: bile pigments
Reddish-brown: hemoglobin
Brown to brown-black: melanin

2. *Odor* is usually not of special diagnostic significance. Normal freshly voided urine is aromatic. On standing, there is an ammonia odor secondary to the decomposition of urea. In a UTI, it *may* be foul-smelling with high bacterial counts. Other alterations in odor include:

Sweet and fruity: diabetes
Fecal odor: contamination
Foods: for example, asparagus, onions

3. *Turbidity* of urine should be clear and transparent. Cloudiness may be secondary to WBCs, bacteria, phosphates, and carbonates. In the UTI, one of the most common causes is alkalinity.

4. *pH* of urine should be acidic. If the urine is highly alkaline, that is, 7.5, think UTI or bacterial contamination. You will need to check for urea splitting organisms, for example, *Proteus* which is associated with recurrent infections and stone formation.

5. *Blood* can be due to hemolysis in the bloodstream, any body organ, as well as the urinary tract. It may also accompany severe infectious disease, poisoning, increased exercise, and burns.

6. *Ketones* are increased in vomiting, diarrhea, dieting.

7. *Glucose* could be due to diabetes mellitus, can follow a heavy high carbohydrate meal, or increased stress.

8. *Bilirubin* may indicate hepatocellular disease, biliary obstruction.

9. *Protein* has little relationship to UTIs. Transient, intermittent protein is usually physiologic or functional (e.g., fever, increased exercise) rather than a renal disorder. Blood and protein in the urine is an important finding; it is quite often due to renal disease.

Microscopic. There is much discussion over the technique involved, for example, centrifuged (spun) versus uncentrifuged (unspun) specimen. Suggested techniques include:

1. Gram's stain smears of uncentrifuged urine (presence of 1 to 2 organisms per one immersion field correlates with bacterial concentration of 10^5 organisms/ml)

2. Centrifuge urine (300 rpm for three minutes). Examine sediment with a coverslip under high dry power. (Presence of ≥ 20 bacteria/HPF correlate with 10^5 organisms/ml)

Looking at the specimen, the nurse practitioner should identify any red blood cells, casts, WBCs, and most importantly, bacteria.

1. *Red blood cells* may be due to trauma, contamination, exercise. They are significant when accompanied by casts, which suggests upper urinary tract infection.

2. *Casts* are classified as to the material they contain:

a. *WBC* casts may be seen in acute glomerulonephritis

b. *RBC* casts may be seen in acute inflammatory or vascular disorders of the glomerulus

c. *Epithelial cell* casts may indicate acute inflammatory disease

d. *Granular* casts may indicate pyelonephritis but can be found in febrile illnesses

e. *Hyaline* casts may indicate damage to the glomerular capillary membrane, however, can also be found in normal children

3. *Pyuria* is the presence of pus cells (polymorphonuclear leukocytes) in the urine. It is not a reliable predictor of a UTI. The cells may be absent in up to 50% of children with significant bacteriuria. Pyuria is generally considered significant at > 5 to 10 WBCs/HPF per centrifuged specimen. Other causes of pyuria include vulvovaginal contaminants, extreme dehydration, appendicitis, and poor hygiene. If a significant number of WBCs is seen without bacteria, a urine culture should be obtained before initiating treatment.

4. *Bacteriuria.* The absence of visible bacteria under the microscope does not always mean that the urine is sterile. They may be decreased, for example, due to dilute urine, increased acidity of urine, or medication. The diagnosis of a UTI is, however, based on the finding of a significant growth

of bacteria from a urine culture. As noted previously, the majority of cases are due to *E. coli* followed by *Klebsiella, Proteus mirabilis, Enterobacter, Staphylococcus epidermidis, enterococcus,* or *Pseudomonas.*

Ideally, two consecutive (obtained a few days apart) clean-catch specimens with $\geq 10^5$ organisms should be obtained. This often is not feasible, however. In the symptomatic child, a single urine culture with $>10^5$ organisms (same species) correlates with an 80% likelihood of infection; two consecutive positive cultures is 96%. Lower counts (10,000 to 100,000 organisms/ml) may mean infection, especially in those children with past UTIs. Less than 10,000 organisms is usually the result of a contaminant.

Management

The nurse practitioner should seek medical consultation upon diagnosis of a UTI in the infant and young child. The aim of the management of UTIs in children is to eradicate acute infection and to decrease recurrence. The early detection of correctable abnormalities is essential. It must be noted that the prognosis for long-term morbidity and mortality is not known, whether there is pharmacologic treatment or not. Seventy-five percent of children who are adequately treated for uncomplicated UTIs have recurrences within 18 months. Fifty to 65% of these recurrences are asymptomatic, which supports the notion to refer all first infections for radiologic work-up.

There is debate as to when the child should have an intravenous pyelogram (IVP) and a voiding cystourethrogram (VCUG). The structure of the urinary tract needs to be assessed to rule out anomalies including obstruction. It is safest to refer all children with UTIs for evaluation once their infection has cleared. If these are normal, the child should be followed with urine cultures for at least two years, that is, every month for the first 3 months, every 3 months for the next 9 months, every 6 months for the last 12 months.

Counseling. The caregiver needs reassurance that with proper treatment the child with an uncomplicated UTI will do well. They should be instructed to examine the urine and note any characteristics out of the normal. Periodic home-testing of a freshly voided sample may be valuable. There are several commercial, inexpensive culture and chemical methods available, for example, Dip-slide and the Microstix dip-strip nitrite test. (Dietary nitrate is reduced to nitrite by enteric gram-negative bacteria.)

Good hygiene is essential. Girls need to be taught to wipe from front to back. Bubble baths should be avoided. Large, constipated stools can be avoided with dietary management and increased fluids. The child should be encouraged to void frequently with complete emptying. Cotton underpants should be worn. If the child is found scratching the perianal area, he or she should be checked for pinworms.

Pharmacology. Antibacterial agents are selected on the basis of sensitivity testing. If the child has WBCs plus bacteria, treatment is most often begun before the culture results are available.

In uncomplicated UTIs, the sulfonamides are a first-line medication; they are one of the least expensive and most effective. They also have fewer gastrointestinal side effects than do antibiotics.

Within 48 hours, the urine should be sterile. If possible, the urine should be cultured on day three of treatment to assure the efficacy of the drug, and again one week post treatment.

Recently, studies have supported the use of one-dose or few-day treatment with antimicrobials. This is usually effective with lower tract infections. However, treatment for 10 to 14 days is generally recommended (see Table 11.1).

Trimethoprim-sulfamethoxazole and nitrofurantoin are commonly used prophylactically in frequent recurrences of UTIs. They produce fewer resistant organisms in the intestinal flora. The usual dose is 1 tablet daily at bedtime.

Referral. A medical health care provider should be consulted before treatment is initiated, especially for the infant and younger child. Referral is indicated if the child is still symptomatic after being on the medication for two to three days; if the microscopic examination of the urine continues to reveal bacteria; or, if the follow-up urine culture is not sterile.

If the nurse practitioner/physician have managed the child to the point of radiographic studies, a referral to a urologist is indicated if the roentgenogram shows obstruction or severe reflux. Reflux often disappears as children get older; however, severe reflux compromised by persistent infection has a poorer prognosis without surgical intervention.

Table 11.1. Common Therapeutic Agents

Drug	Dosage	Considerations
Sulfisoxazole (Gantrisin)	100 to 150 mg/kg/d in 4 divided doses	Avoid in third trimester of pregnancy, newborns, infants, and G-6PD-deficient children
Ampicillin/amoxicillin	50 to 100 mg/kg/d in 4 divided doses	Preferred in pregnancy
Trimethoprim-sulfamethoxazole (Septra, Bactrim)	8 mg/kg/d trimethoprim plus 40 mg/kg/d sulfamethoxazole in 2 divided doses	Avoid in pregnancy, newborns, and G-6PD-deficient children
Nitrofurantoin (Furadantin)	5 to 7 mg/kg/d in 4 divided doses	Avoid in pregnancy, newborns, and G-6PD-deficient children
Cephalexin or cephradine (Velosef, Anspor)	25 to 50 mg/kg/d in 4 divided doses	Preferred in pregnancy

ASYMPTOMATIC UTIs

The significance of asymptomatic bacteriuria (ABU) is not clear; however, it is an abnormal finding. In premature newborns, the prevalence is about 3%; at term, 1%. Preschool children have an incidence of between 1 and 1.5%; school ages, 1.5%. Girls are at greater risk at all ages except the newborn period.

Asymptomatic bacteriuria is found in children coincidentally through screening programs. Those at risk are females (20 females: 1 male), children under 5 (there is less scarring after that time), premature infants, and pregnant women.

HISTORY

Upon discovery of the bacteriuria, a thorough history needs to be obtained (see symptomatic UTIs).

PHYSICAL EXAMINATION

A complete examination should be accomplished (see symptomatic UTIs).

DIAGNOSTIC TESTS

Screening for bacteriuria requires *three* consecutive cultures that are positive at $\geq 10^5$ organisms (same species). If this is not accomplished, there is a real potential for overdiagnosis. Otherwise, the same procedures may be utilized as with symptomatic UTIs.

MANAGEMENT

Early detection and treatment is not shown to prevent progressive disease. Anatomical abnormalities and obstructions, however, have been identified by intravenous pyelogram (IVP) and voiding cystourethrograms (VCUG) in as many as 30% of children with ABU.

Counseling

(See symptomatic urinary tract counseling.)

Pharmacology

There is considerable discussion over the use of antimicrobial agents. It is generally agreed to treat these children the same as those with symptomatic UTIs.

Referral

As with symptomatic UTIs, consultation should be solicited when treating the infant and younger child. Referral is indicated if the child becomes symptomatic during treatment, if the microscopic examination of the urine reveals bacteria and/or if the follow-up urine culture is not sterile. If the nurse practitioner/physician find abnormalities on radiographic studies, a referral to a urologist is indicated.

STUDY QUESTIONS

Circle all that apply .

Mrs. Smith brings 2-month-old John to your clinic. He has been very irritable with a rectal temperature of 101°F. On history, you find he has had occasional diarrheal stools with frequent damp diapers in between.

1. Further indicator(s) of a UTI would include:

   a. clean-catch bagged urine with ≤ 3 bacteria/HPF (spun)
   b. suprapubic aspiration with 10 bacteria/HPF (unspun Gram's stain)
   c. dark yellow urine
   d. >10 WBCs/HPF (spun)

2. The diagnosis of a UTI is confirmed. Your next step(s) is/are:

   a. do urine culture
   b. begin ampicillin 50 mg/kg/d in 4 divided doses for 10 to 14 days
   c. refer to physician as the UTI may quickly lead to scarring
   d. schedule IVP, voiding cystourethrogram

3. Mrs. Clark brings 4-year-old Susan to your clinic. Susan has been complaining of dysuria, enuresis (which she has not had previously) and occasional constipation. She has never had a UTI before. Other symptoms of a UTI that you might expect in this age group include:

    a. trouble starting flow
    b. abdominal pain
    c. dribbling
    d. fever

4. Susan has also been found by her mother to have perineal itching and a slight vaginal discharge. Your differential diagnosis would include:

    a. streptococcal vaginitis
    b. foreign body
    c. pinworms
    d. poor hygiene

5. Your physical examination is unremarkable with the exception of mild perineal irritation due to soap and powder residue. *You* obtain a clean-catch midstream urine. The urinalysis reveals milky-colored urine, trace protein, pH of 8. This could indicate:

    a. pus cells in the urine
    b. probably normal protein
    c. alkaline urine, may be *Proteus*
    d. vaginal contamination

6. Your microscopic examination on a spun specimen reveals 10 WBCs, 30 to 40 rods/HPF. Your diagnostic tests/management at this point include:

    a. hold treatment until C&S results are back
    b. do urine for C&S
    c. schedule IVP, VCUG within next 10 days
    d. begin sulfisoxazole 100 mgm/kg/d in 4 divided doses x 10 days

7. Your instructions to Mrs. Clark include:

    a. bring Susan back to the clinic in three days for a follow-up urine culture to see if the medication is working
    b. have Susan drink plenty of liquids, especially water, to help prevent constipation
    c. assist Susan with her bath/shower; encourage her to wipe front to back after going to the bathroom
    d. Susan will probably need medication every night to prevent a recurrence of this infection

8. You are involved in a screening program at a day care center. You are using a dip-strip nitrite test to detect asymptomatic bacteriuria. This is important in that:

   a. children under 5 have less scarring if there are abnormalities
   b. caregivers can be instructed in home monitoring for bacteriuria
   c. between 1 to 1.5% of preschool children will have asymptomatic bacteriuria
   d. asymptomatic bacteriuria is insignificant; screening is not indicated

9. Beth, a 3½-year-old, is found to have a positive nitrite test. Her mother is concerned that she should begin medication immediately. You reassure her that with proper treatment, Beth will do well. You tell her that Beth's treatment should include:

   a. seeing her private health care provider
   b. sulfonamides for 10 to 14 days
   c. three consecutive positive cultures
   d. radiographic studies

10. You confer with Beth's P.M.D. who confirmed the diagnosis of a UTI. He ordered VCUG that revealed severe vesicoureteral reflux. This supports the notion(s) that

   a. radiographic follow-up is not indicated since reflux often disappears as children get older
   b. the early detection and treatment of asymptomatic bacteriuria is indicated, especially in high risk groups
   c. prophylactic medications (e.g., nitrofurantoin) are indicated qhs
   d. anatomical abnormalities and obstructions are identified in as many as 30% of children with asymptomatic bacteriuria

ANSWERS

1. b, d	6. b, d
2. a, c	7. a, b, c
3. b, d	8. a, b, c
4. a, b, c, d	9. a, c
5. a, b, c	10. b, d

BIBLIOGRAPHY

Kay, D. How to diagnose and treat urinary tract infections. *Medical Times,* March, 1981, 59–63.

King, L. R. Bacterial infections of the urinary tract (female children), in Conn, H. F. (Ed.): *1981 Current Therapy.* Philadelphia: W. B. Saunders, 1981.

Kunin, C. M. *Detection, prevention and management of urinary tract infections.* (3rd. ed.). Philadelphia: Lea and Febiger, 1979.

McCoy, J. A. Preliminary diagnosis of urinary tract infection in symptomatic children. *The Nurse Practitioner,* January 1982, 7, 1, 23–33, 48.

Monahan, M., & Resnick, J. Urinary tract infections in girls: age at onset and urinary tract abnormalities. *Pediatrics,* August 1978, 62, 2, 237–239.

Rapkin, R. H. Urinary tract infection in childhood. *Pediatrics,* October 1977, 60, 4, 508–511.

CHAPTER **12**

SKIN DISORDERS

Terry E. Tippett Neilson
Pamela K. Busher

The primary care provider is often called upon to manage initial skin rashes or minor skin disorders. Given the myriad dermatologic problems possible, the nurse practitioner can best direct his or her efforts by systematically examining the skin and then appropriately classifying the primary and secondary lesions. The additional compilation of a chronologic history of the disorder, patient medical-pharmacology history, and social-occupational history will further guide the practitioner toward the decision to treat or refer the client. The basis for a practitioner's dermatologic assessment will usually rest on clinical and historical impressions. Elaborate definitive laboratory tests are not usually available in primary care settings and are mentioned for informative purposes.

DIAPER RASH

Very few babies, if any, have passed through the diaper stage without a rash. During this period, a child's bottom may come in contact with a variety of commercial soaps, disposable diapers, plastic pants, and various lotions, as well as intestinal organisms and urine.

Most diaper rashes respond quickly to frequent changing and cleaning, while others persist regardless of meticulous care. However, prevention of diaper rashes is far more important than treatment. Educating the parents on the following preventive measures is essential:

1. Change diapers frequently
2. Use synthetic liners with cloth diapers since liners tend to decrease the contact of the skin to urine; disposable diapers have synthetic linings
3. Rinse and dry diapered area with every change
4. After fecal soiling, cleanse diapered area with mineral oil or cottonseed oil instead of water
5. Avoid tight-fitting waterproof pants; they confine the concentrated ammonia in the diapered area
6. At the first signs of erythema, apply a protective ointment (e.g., zinc oxide or Vaseline jelly)
7. Use a mild detergent to wash diapers and double rinse to remove all soap

AMMONIA DIAPER RASH

Most diaper rash is caused by direct contact of the skin to ammonia that is formed in voided urine. It is more difficult to control the rash in warm humid climates.

Physical Examination

Diaper rash is an erythematous and papulovesicular dermatitis. It is located on the thighs, genitals, lower abdomen, and the convex surfaces of the buttock. The skin folds in the diapered area are unaffected as they do not come in direct contact with the urine.

Management

Explain the cause of the rash to the parents. Encourage them to expose the baby's diapered area to warm dry air (heat-lamp, sun) for at least 30 minutes four times a day. Initiate the preventive measures outlined previously.

CANDIDA DIAPER RASH

Some infants carry *Candida albicans* in their gastrointestinal tract and are predisposed to this type of diaper rash. The *C. albicans* flourish in the warm moist environment of the diaper. It is a very frustrating rash as it tends to recur.

Physical Examination

The *Candida* rash produces an intensely erythematous, confluent plague with nearby satellite red macules or vesicopustules. It differs from the ammonia rash since it is often located in the inguinal folds and perirectal skin. The perineum and lower abdomen may also be involved. Oral thrush may be present.

Management

Initiate the general preventive measures. An anticandida agent (nystatin, miconazole, and amphotericin B) in ointment form should be applied to the diaper area with every change. If inflammation is severe, a nonfluorinated corticosteroid ointment may be used. When recurrences are frequent, an oral anticandida agent is necessary.

BACTERIAL DIAPER RASH

A primary bacterial diaper rash is due to poor hygiene. The organism most responsible is *E. coli*. When the diapered area is inadequately cleaned and dried, fecal soil and debris accumulate in the folds of the groin. The bacteria has the perfect environment to replicate. The heavier the child and the warmer the climate, the greater the problem

With a preexisting diaper rash, the intestinal bacteria can produce a secondary infection. This mixed diaper rash can be challenging to treat.

Physical Examination

The bacterial diaper rash is an erythematous pustular dermatitis. Similar to the rash of *Candida,* the bacterial diaper rash is first seen in the inguinal folds and the perirectal skin. Unlike the *Candida* rash, it has no satellite lesions. If poor hygiene is the problem, it is not uncommon for the intertriginous areas of the neck and axilla to be involved as well.

Management

As with all diaper rashes, it is essential to initiate the general preventive measures. The affected areas should be washed with an antibacterial soap (Dial, Safeguard) and dried thoroughly. Apply an unscented talc powder and topical antibiotic ointment about three or four times daily. If it is a mixed diaper rash, a combination ointment such as Mycolog (nystatin-neomycin-gramicidin-triamcinolone) is frequently used.

SEBORRHEIC DERMATITIS
(CRADLE CAP)

Although it appears as dry skin, cradle cap is actually very oily. Many texts refer to seborrheic conditions as the result of a basic defect in an oil gland leaking under the skin. However, the cause is not known and, although the disorder is controllable, it is not curable. It is an inherited condition in some.

Most newborn's skin is washed and oiled daily. Frequently, first-time parents avoid washing the infant's head, especially over the soft spots. They fear they will cause damage to the baby's brain. Since cradle cap looks like dry skin, the inexperienced parent will often lubricate the head along with the rest of the newborn's skin.

PHYSICAL EXAMINATION

Lesions are yellowish, greasy, scaly, red, papulosquamous patches. The scalp is most frequently involved. However, eyebrows, nasolabial areas, and post-auricular regions are involved in more extensive cases.

MANAGEMENT

It is important that the parents have a sound understanding of the causes. Stress that the skin is oily, not dry, and washing the soft spots will not hurt the baby. Encourage daily washing of the scalp and affected area with a mild shampoo. While shampooing, gently scratch the scales with fingernails to loosen them. After shampooing, comb hair with a fine-tooth comb to remove as much of the scales as possible.

Topical steroids are reserved for the more severe cases. The steroids reduce inflammation and shedding of skin.

ATOPIC DERMATITIS
(ECZEMA)

Atopic dermatitis is one of the most common as well as one of the most perplexing and difficult skin conditions to manage. It is a chronic, pruritic, superficial inflammation (dry skin) usually found in people with a personal or family history of allergic disorders (asthma, atopic dermatitis, hay fever, or urticaria). Atopic dermatitis is more common in infants and young children than in adults and most outgrow it by age 5. Nearly 30% of children with atopic dermatitis develop hay fever or asthma.

During the winter months, atopic dermatitis tends to become more of a problem. This is because most home heating systems produce a very dry air that aggravates the already dry skin problem. Also, wool products are worn more in the colder months and tend to make this chronic condition worse.

Certain foods, especially with infants and young children, tend to aggravate atopic dermatitis. If these foods can be identified, they should be avoided.

PHYSICAL EXAMINATION

Acute manifestations of atopic dermatitis are characterized by erythema, pruritis, and vesicles. These conditions are more common in infants and young children. Adolescents and adults tend to have a more chronic atopic dermatitis. The skin, in the chronic form, is very dry with lichenification, fissuring, and excoriations.

Areas involved vary with the age of the child. In very young infants, the eruptions are found on the scalp, face, ears, neck, trunk, and diaper area. In the older child or adult, the areas involved are primarily the hands and feet as well as the flexor surfaces of the knees, elbows, and wrists.

MANAGEMENT

Counseling

Parent education is essential. Everyone involved in the care of a child with atopic dermatitis needs to have a sound understanding of this skin condition. Education on the following points is essential:

1. This is an inherited disease in which skin tests are usually not helpful. There is no cure, but symptomatic relief of the pruritis and control of the skin manifestations are possible.
2. In the winter months, humidify the air. Basins of water may be placed around the house.
3. Avoid contact with wool and products containing lanolin (wool fat).
4. Encourage the child to follow a regular diet but omit those foods that aggravate the rash.
5. Use bath oils to trap water in the skin. However, avoid excessive bathing, especially during winter months.

Pharmacology

As previously stated, this skin disorder can be controlled but not cured. Topical steroids are used to decrease inflammation. Benadryl is used as a sedative and to decrease the pruritis.

SCABIES

The infestation of the skin, called scabies, is caused by *Sarcoptes scabiei,* a female mite that burrows into the skin, depositing eggs and fecal pellets. In contrast to popular belief, scabies is not common in the general population. School-age children and people living in overcrowded conditions are more likely to contract scabies. However, epidemic outbreaks have occurred in unpredictable patterns. The most recent outbreak occurred in the 1970s.

PHYSICAL EXAMINATION

The initial lesion consists of a small vesicle at the point where the female mite burrowed into the skin. This produces a red, 2 mm linear elevation of the skin. The subsequent skin manifestations consist of scaling, papules, excoriations, and vesicles in a linear pattern (run). Secondary infection is common.

These lesions are seen most frequently in the inguinal area, the axilla, the popliteal folds and the webs of the fingers. Scabies rarely occurs on the face except with nursing infants whose mothers have lesions on the breast. Itching is worse at night.

DIAGNOSTIC TESTS

Since the female *S. scabiei* is not visible to the naked eye, the disease is confirmed by microscopic viewing of the mite. This procedure requires skillful scraping of the burrow.

MANAGEMENT

Counseling

Education of the following points is essential:

1. All family members need to be checked for scabies
2. All bed linen and clothing needs to be completely washed; sterilization is unnecessary

3. Itching may persist for two weeks after treatment; if longer than two weeks, reexamination is required

Pharmacology

Gamma benzene hexachloride (1% in a cream base) is the drug of choice. The cream is applied to the entire body, left on for 24 hours, and completely rinsed off. The treatment is repeated after five days, up to three times.

PYOGENIC BACTERIAL INFECTION

Coagulase-positive staphylococci and, occasionally, beta-hemolytic streptococci are the common causative agents of superficial bacterial skin infections. This section will discuss impetigo, folliculitis, furuncles, and carbuncles.

Generally, people do not go to health care providers for a single bacterial lesion of the skin, however, they do seek advice for several lesions or recurring lesions. In clients with recurring bacterial skin infections, especially furuncles (boils), diabetes must be eliminated as a cause of the infection.

Client education is the key for a rapid recovery and prevention of future bacterial infections. In managing clients with pyodermas, three general counseling principles should be discussed.

1. *Bathing.* Frequent bathing with bactericidal soaps (Dial, Safeguard) is necessary. Encourage the removal of crusts from the lesions during bathing to facilitate penetration of the medication.
2. *Isolation.* Linens and clothing should be cleaned frequently. The client should have a separate washcloth and towel. Hand washing should be stressed.
3. *Diet.* Fatty foods (chocolate, nuts, and dairy products) should be avoided in those clients with recurring bacterial skin infections (1).

IMPETIGO

Impetigo is an extremely contagious skin disease in infants and young children. In adults and older children, the disease is seen less frequently and does not appear to be as contagious. Coagulase-positive staphylococci and occasionally beta-hemolytic streptococci are the causative organisms. Predisposing factors are poor health and poor hygiene.

Physical Examination

Impetigo is most common on the extremities and the face. It is characterized by honey-colored "stuck-on" crusts which follow the rupture of preceding vesicles, bullae, and pustules. The crusts are surrounded by erythematous skin. Bullae are common in infants and young children.

Management

Counseling. Cleanliness is most important. Counseling the parent on frequent bathing with a bactericidal soap and general isolation principles is essential. Wet dressings to soak the crusts may be necessary before they can be removed.

Pharmacology. Either topical antibiotic preparations (combinations of bacitracin, neomycin, and polymycin) or systemic antibiotics need to be initiated. Since the risk of glomerulonephritis exists, many practitioners question the use of topical antibiotics in the treatment of impetigo.

FOLLICULITIS, FURUNCLES, AND CARBUNCLES

Folliculitis, furuncles, and carbuncles are infections of hair follicles and are usually caused by coagulase-positive staphylococci. Folliculitis and furuncles involve only one hair follicle while carbuncles involve several. Both furuncles (boils) and carbuncles are considered a more extensive infection than folliculitis. Some predisposing factors to these infections are poor hygiene, obesity, diabetes, and diets rich in sugars and fats.

PHYSICAL EXAMINATION

Folliculitis is a single pustule or papule originating within a hair follicle. It is seen most often on the scalp, face, buttocks, and the extensor surfaces of extremities.

A furuncle or carbuncle starts as a red, hard, tender, hot nodule which breaks down to form a necrotic core with a pustular point. The most common sites are the posterior neck and buttocks.

MANAGEMENT

Counseling

Initiate the three general counseling principles outlined in the beginning of this section. It is important to educate the clients never to squeeze these lesions. Occasionally, septicemia occurs from squeezing. Apply hot compresses to the affected area three times daily. Referral for incision and drainage may be necessary for furuncles and carbuncles if fluctuation is noted.

Pharmacology

A systemic antibiotic (penicillin is the drug of choice) is usually indicated only for furuncles and carbuncles. However, with recurring folliculitis, systemic antibiotics are useful.

TINEA

Tinea is a broad term that includes superficial skin infections caused by three genera of fungi: *Trichophyton, Epidermophyton,* and *Microsporum.* Tinea infections are very common in humans.

To confirm a fungal infection, skin scrapings are taken from the active border of the lesion, placed on a microscope slide, covered with 20% aqueous potassium hydroxide solution (KOH), and a cover slip. The slide is heated briefly or allowed to stand for 30 minutes. The KOH solution dissolves the skin and allows the fungi to be viewed easily under the microscope as branched hyphae (threadlike, branching filaments). The Wood's light is an easy method of diagnosing tinea infection from the *Microsporum* genus. Under a Wood's light, hairs or skin infected with this class of fungus will fluoresce with a bright yellowish-green color. Culture is necessary for accurate identification of all species but is not cost effective.

TINEA CAPITIS

Tinea capitis is the most common cause of hair loss among children 3 to 8 years of age. It is uncommon in adults, probably because they have less contact with animals than young children. Cats and dogs are the most frequent carriers of the fungus. Occasionally, it may be transmitted from person to person.

History and Physical Examination

Although the lesions may appear anywhere on the scalp, they are most frequently located on the occipital area. They are described as rounded bald spots with varying degrees of inflammation. Classically, small broken-off hairs can be seen in the lesion.

Diagnostic Tests

Since 90% or greater of all tinea capitis is due to the class of fungus called *Microsporum*, examination of the scalp with a Wood's light is recommended. Skin scrapings in KOH solution are also useful.

Management

Counseling. Be sure your clients understand that tinea capitis is spread by household pets (especially kittens and puppies) and less frequently by humans. Therefore, treatment is encouraged for all afflicted family members and pets. Advise against the exchange of head gear. Encourage follow-up visits to determine care.

Clip the hair closely in the vicinity of the lesion. Gently scrub the scalp with a synthetic nonfat soap. This will help to prevent secondary infections.

Pharmacology. The treatment of choice is oral griseofulvin 20 mg/kg/24 hours in three doses for four to eight weeks. Signs of healing should be visible by the third week of treatment.

TINEA CORPORIS (RINGWORM)

Ringworm can be caused by any of the dermatophytes; however, the animal-borne *Microsporum* class is responsible for most cases. It is seen more frequently in children than adults because children are more likely to have close contact with animals, especially kittens and puppies. It also can be spread from person to person. The incidence is higher in warm humid areas.

Physical Examination

Tinea corporis is a gradually expanding erythematous ring. Its elevated margins contain scales and pinpoint vesicles. The center of the ring heals as its circumference enlarges. It is found most often on the forearms, hands, neck, and face, but any part of the body may be involved. Itching is very mild.

Management

Counseling. Explain that ringworm is spread by close contact with household pets and occasionally by contact with another person who has an active tinea corporis infection. Therefore, all family members and pets need to be checked for tinea. Avoid exchanging clothing without adequate laundering.

Pharmacology. For small patches of ringworm, topical antifungal agents are used (tolnaftate, clotrimazole, or haloprogin). If the area of involvement is extensive or recurring, the drug of choice is oral griseofulvin for three to six weeks or until the lesions have healed.

TINEA CRURIS (JOCK ITCH)

Tinea cruris frequently occurs concurrently with athlete's foot. It is believed to be spread from the feet because people tend to dry their feet before their groin after bathing. Tinea cruris is not very contagious, even between husband and wife. Men appear to be more susceptible to the infection.

Physical Examination

Lesions are scaly, red plaques, which are sharply circumscribed with pinpoint vesicles on the border. There is a tendency for central healing; however, the clinical appearance may be altered by perspiration and secondary infections. Lesions are very common during adolescence, especially in the inguinal area.

Management

Counseling. Special emphasis needs to be placed on personal hygiene. After bathing, educate clients to dry their feet last. When perspiring excessively, advise dusting powder or cornstarch on the involved area two or three times daily.

Pharmacology. If the involved area is small, an antifungal cream (tolnaftate, clotrimazole or haloprogin) should be applied to the area three times daily. For more extensive cases, oral griseofulvin for six to eight weeks is recommended.

TINEA PEDIS (ATHLETE'S FOOT)

Superficial fungus infections of the feet, probably very widespread in older children and adults, do not always produce clinical manifestations. It is difficult to cure tinea pedis and if the toenails are involved, a cure is unlikely.

Contrary to popular opinion, athlete's foot is not very contagious. Men are affected much more than women. It is believed that there is a susceptibility factor necessary for infection.

Physical Examination

Early signs include scaling, maceration, and fissuring of the toe webs. These may extend to the sole as patchy red, scaling and deep-seated vesicles. The fourth web space is most commonly involved. Bacterial complications are common.

Management

Counseling.   Client education needs to focus on personal hygiene. The following points are important:

1. After bathing, dry carefully between toes and dry feet last
2. Wear wooden sandals in community showers and bathing places
3. Wear well-ventilated shoes
4. Change socks frequently (white socks are unnecessary)
5. Stress that this is a chronic condition and is difficult to cure

Pharmacology.   Apply topical antifungal ointments to the involved areas three times daily. Blisters should be drained and trimmed so the medication can reach the fungus. Examples of antifungal agents are tolnaftate, clotrimazole, and haloprogin.

TINEA VERSICOLOR

Tinea versicolor is a noninflammatory fungal infection. It acquired its name from the varying color of its lesions. On a sun-tanned person, the lesions are pale or white; however, on fair skin, the lesions are tan—they 'versi' (turn) color. The lesions are primarily of cosmetic concern and are not symptomatic.

Physical Examination

The lesions are papulosquamous or maculosquamous patches of varying size and shape. Since these lesions do not tan, they are more obvious during the summer.

Management

Advise clients to bathe and dry thoroughly. Apply Selsun lotion over the entire body, leave it on for 24 hours, and then rinse completely. Repeat this procedure weekly for four treatments.

CONTACT DERMATITIS

This common inflammatory reaction can result from direct or indirect skin contact with a specific irritant or allergen. Common irritants include solvents, acids, soaps, oils, polishes, and bleaches. Usual allergens include cosmetics, topical pharmacologic preparations, rubber products, and plant resins. The most common contact dermatitis seen by the primary care provider is that resulting from poison oak or poison ivy. Initial incubation after exposure ranges from days to weeks; reexposure incubation lasts from 12 to 48 hours.

HISTORY AND PHYSICAL EXAMINATION

The client should be questioned for new or recent exposure to topical medications, cosmetics, new clothing fabrics, soaps, and plants. Pets can carry the resin of plants on their bodies and the smoke of burning plants can carry the irritant. Occupations, hobbies, and recent outdoor activities should be carefully screened for. Physical exam will reveal early erythematous areas quickly erupting into pruritic vesicles. Plant contact often leaves revealing linear streaks of erythematous vesicles where the plant brushed against the skin.

MANAGEMENT

The goal of treatment is to identify and remove the contact agent and to treat the inflammation.

1. Wet, oozing lesions can be dried with soaks of Burow's solution (1:20) four to six times a day.
2. Colloidal oatmeal baths can provide relief as well as drying properties.
3. Antipruritic therapy is appropriate every four to six hours as well as at bedtime (e.g., Benadryl or Periactin).
4. Antiinflammatory creams, such as fluorinated steroids are appropriate for short-term use.

Counseling

Client education should focus on avoidance of the known contact agent. If no agent is identified the client should avoid such potential agents as abrasive soaps, detergents, solvents, and bleaches. Hypoallergenic cosmetics should be used and the client should wash thoroughly after work or outdoor activities.

Referral

Bullous eruptions should be referred for systemic steroid treatment.

HERPES VIRUS HOMINUS (HVH)

This large DNA virus has two distinct antiogenic strains: type I associated with lesions above the umbilicus, and type II occurring below the umbilicus. The strains can, however, be cross-transferred. Entrance of this virus into the body may cause a clinical or subclinical infection. After the initial infection, it is believed the virus travels up a local nerve axon where it remains in a latent state in the regional ganglia. The virus can be periodically reactivated and conducted to the skin via peripheral nerve fibers where it again replicates on the skin. There are two forms to both strains: (1) the painful primary infection and (2) the less severe recurrent or secondary infection.

HERPES SIMPLEX (TYPE I)

Herpes simplex, or the nongenital form, is a benign viral infection. The virus is believed to be transmittable until new pink skin appears on the lesions.

History and Physical Examination

The primary infection usually appears as a gingivostomatitis lasting one to three weeks. A prodrome of local tenderness can precede the clinical infection for a day or two after which the client complains of an outbreak of extremely painful lesions, localized lymphadenopathy, fever, and malaise. The vesicles appear as grouped, clear lesions on an erythematous base. After several days they become turbid and coalesce. This is followed by crust formation for four to eight days. Children may experience the most dramatic symptoms with fevers up to 105°F., a dramatic increase in salivation, and difficulty eating and drinking that can lead to dehydration. A purulent malodorous drainage may accompany the lesions and can extend over the entire buccal mucosa.

The secondary or recurrent form is less acute and lasts for only seven to ten days. There is usually no systemic component. Signs and symptoms include localized lymphadenopathy and moderate paresthesias from nerve irritation. The lesions are less painful, but again may be preceded by a prodrome of tingling, burning, and itching hours to days before the actual outbreak. The recurrent infection does not commonly occur in the oral cavity, but can appear periodically on the cheeks, nose, neck, anogenital area, sacrum, and buttocks.

Diagnostic Tests

The diagnosis is essentially made from clinical signs, but can be confirmed via culture, skin biopsy, cytologic smear, or antibody titer.

Management

Counseling. Since herpes is a virus, treatment is symptomatic. Saline mouthwash and gargles may soothe tender mucosa. Encourage fluids but caution clients to avoid citrus and carbonated drinks. All clients should isolate themselves from newborns and immunosuppressed people. Attention to prevention can be of help by minimizing precipitants, such as sunlight, psychologic stress, colds, fever, and menstrual tensions.

Pharmacology (Primary Infection). The goal is to control pain and to prevent secondary infections:

1. Salicylates or acetaminophen for analgesia; if not effective, consult with physician about providing narcotics for two weeks
2. Xylocaine jelly may be applied as needed for topical anesthesia

3. Cleansing mouthwashes of Zephiran 1:1000 or tetracycline suspension may reduce secondary infection
4. Healing time may be reduced in some clients with the use of topical anti-viral agents (e.g., Stoxil)

Since the secondary or recurrent form of herpes is less painful, has a shorter duration, and causes less of a systemic reaction, it is more of a cosmetic concern to the client.

1. Apply drying agents (e.g. Blistex, Camphophenique, 10% aluminum acetate)
2. Prescribe topical antibiotics for secondary bacterial infections

HERPES SIMPLEX (TYPE II)

The herpes Type II virus, which affects mucous membranes below the umbilicus, is one of the most common of the sexually-transmitted diseases. Close contact with an infected person can also cause infection. There is no cure, and treatment is primarily symptomatic. The incubation period can range from two to ten days with the course lasting from three to six weeks. Like the type I disorder, the type II virus remains in a latent state after the primary infection, in this case, in cells in the area of the original lesion. Most clients affected are beyond the age of puberty and women affected have a five to ten times greater incidence of cervical dysplasia and carcinoma. Newborns delivered vaginally during an infection in the mother can contract a disseminated form of the disease—often with fatal consequences.

History and Physical Exam

The client is sexually active, often has multiple partners, and may give a history of recent known exposure. Men and women are affected equally. The medical history often reveals previous herpetic infections in the genital area. The client may complain of a prodrome of mild paresthesias or burning in any of the following areas: vulvar, genitocrural folds, perianal, vaginal mucosa, urethral meatus, and external penis. Primary infection causes much more severe symptoms than a recurrent infection. With a recurrent infection, the client may have a recent history of fever, emotional stress, or recent menstruation. The lesions are found in the same location as the primary case.

In the acute form, the client complains of continuous, often severe, vulvar or penile pain, dysuria, urinary retention, dyspareunia, itching, fever, headache, and/or malaise. Upon physical exam, the client may show restricted ambulatory movement during the initial infection. The lesions consist of indurated papules or vesicles on erythematous bases that often coalesce to form large ulcers. Maceration may occur in moist areas and edema may be present with extensive involvement. Inguinal adenopathy can occur as well.

Diagnostic Tests

Same as for herpes simplex.

Management

Counseling. The client should be educated in the nature of the disease, its transmission, and possible consequences. Sexual activity should be avoided during an outbreak, the client should be carefully monitored during the last trimester of pregnancy, and women should be followed with yearly pap smears because of increased cancer risk.

Pharmacology. Analgesia with acetominophen (Tylenol) or aspirin may or may not be effective. Consideration of narcotic analgesia in consultation with a physician is appropriate. A topical anesthetic such as Nupercaine may be helpful, but the client should be warned to watch for signs of allergic reactions. Acyclovir ointment 5% (Zovirax) is used in primary infections. It is applied every three to four hours, six times a day for seven days.

Referral. Clients should be referred if the infection occurs late in pregnancy, if the primary infection is severe (e.g. if the client is unable to void), or if a secondary bacterial infection occurs.

VERRUCAE (WARTS)

Warts are viral epidermal infections that are transmitted by direct contact or by autoinoculation. Some may resolve spontaneously (probably by an immunologic mechanism), while others remain resistant to treatment. Warts are common in children and young adults. The nurse practitioner needs to differentiate suspicious lesions from corns, calluses, and melanomas.

VERRUS VULGARIS (COMMON WARTS)

Physical Examination

Common warts are usually asymptomatic and may appear anywhere on the skin, especially on the hands, elbows, knees, and periungual areas. Physical exam reveals small, circular, skin-colored to gray-brown papillomas.

Management

Treatment includes dessication and curettage, cryosurgery with liquid nitrogen, or painting with a keratolytic agent or acids.

PLANTAR WARTS

History and Physical Exam

Plantar growths are flat or slightly raised and may appear as single lesions or in groups. They resemble corns and calluses. The client may complain of severe pain upon walking or standing.

Diagnostic Tests

To differentiate between a corn or callus and a wart, shave off the top of the growth. If minute black pinpoint areas of bleeding are found the growth is a wart.

Management

Plantar warts are difficult to treat. The techniques of removal are the same as those for the common wart. The most common treatment is to pare down the thickened skin with a scalpel and then to apply dichloroacetic acid (50 to 80%) to the wart. The treatment can be repeated every one to two weeks.

VERRUCA PLANSE (FLAT WARTS)

Physical Examination

Seen mainly on the dorsa of hands and feet, these multiple small flat growths are slightly pigmented and can appear in linear streaks.

Management

Treatment consists of dessication and curettage or cryotherapy. Flat warts are highly resistant to treatment.

CONDYLOMATA ACUMINATA (VENEREAL WARTS)

Physical Examination

Venereal warts are sexually transmitted and are found on the foreskin, penis, perineum, and vaginal mucosa. They appear as multiple, fleshy, small cauliflower-like papillomas. An offensive-smelling secretion may cover them.

Management

Treatment of choice consists of painting the warts with a mixture of po-
dophyllin resin in tincture of benzoin. The initial treatment should be applied
for one hour then washed off by the client. Weekly treatments can be left on
for up to four hours before washing, depending on the initial response. Surrounding areas of mucosa may be coated with a protective coating. Inform
the client that the lesions may become painful for a few days after treatment.
Any coexisting vaginitis will prolong the course and must be treated. Refer
the client with large numbers of warts, warts on the face, warts on or in the
anus, and resistance to treatment.

STUDY QUESTIONS

Circle all that apply.

1. A very obese 5-month-old infant boy has an erythematous pustular rash
   in the axillae, diaper area, and neck folds. What are the most probable
   causes of the rash?

   a. poor hygiene
   b. obesity
   c. allergy to dairy products
   d. perspiration

2. A 16-year-old boy has had a chronic papulovesicular scaly rash on
   both feet for the past six months. He has tried all the over-the-counter
   preparations for athlete's foot with little success. He has difficulty going
   to sleep at night because his feet itch so much. Your counseling
   includes:

   a. athlete's foot can be controlled but is difficult to cure
   b. he should keep his feet dry and wear well-ventilated shoes
   c. he should change his socks frequently and wear white socks only
   d. after bathing, he should dry his feet last

3. Which of the following are true statements regarding a candida diaper
   rash?

   a. satellite red macules or vesiculopustules are common
   b. the rash is more prevalent in the inguinal folds
   c. the rash is less prevalent in the inguinal folds
   d. it is very easy to cure a candida diaper rash

4. Seven-year-old Tommy has a scaly, papulovesicular rash between his fingers and under his arms. There are several excoriations in a linear pattern. Itching is intense, especially at night. The best assessment is:

   a. contact dermatitis
   b. tinea
   c. atopic dermatitis
   d. scabies

5. Based on your answer in question number 4, which of the following responses would be useful counseling information for Tommy's mother?

   a. avoid exchanging clothes with other children
   b. try using a milder soap
   c. wash all clothes and bed linen
   d. avoid wool and lanolin products

6. Mary, an 8-month old infant, has an erythematous vesicular dermatitis on her face, scalp, and neck. Her mother says that she is always pulling at her rash. There is a strong family history of asthma and chronic skin rashes. The best assessment is:

   a. contact dermatitus
   b. tinea
   c. atopic dermatitis
   d. scabies

7. Based on your answers in question number 6, which of the following responses would be useful counseling information for Mary's mother?

   a. avoid exchanging clothes with other children
   b. try using a milder soap
   c. wash all clothes and bed linen
   d. avoid wool and lanolin products

8. Susie, a six-year-old, has an extensive case of impetigo on her face, arms, and legs. The management of Susie should include:

   a. emphasize the removal of the impetigo's crusts during bathing with Dial soap
   b. use only topical antibiotics to avoid an allergic reaction to penicillin
   c. use a systemic antibiotic (e.g., penicillin or erythromycin)
   d. wash all clothes and bed linen frequently

9. The major complication(s) of impetigo is(are):

   a. rheumatic fever
   b. rheumatoid arthritis
   c. acute glomerulonephritis
   d. hemolytic anemia

10. Management of cradle cap include(s):

    a. shampooing the infant's scalp daily
    b. applying mineral oil to scalp twice a day
    c. topical antibiotics three times a day
    d. gentle removal of scales with a comb

11. To differentiate between a plantar wart and a callus, one would:

    a. apply podophyllin 25% to the lesion; if it is a plantar wart, it should
       shrink in size in 7 days
    b. shave the top of the lesion; if it is a plantar wart, there will be bleed-
       ing points visible on the shaved portion
    c. apply podophyllin 25% to the lesion; if it is a callus, it should shrink in
       size in 7 days
    d. shave the top of the lesion; if it is a callus, there will be bleeding
       points visible on the shaved portion

ANSWERS

1. a, b, d	7. b, d
2. a, b, d	8. a, c, d
3. a, b	9. c
4. d	10. a, d
5. a, c	11. b
6. c	

REFERENCES

1. Sauer, G. C. *Manual of Skin Diseases*, 4th ed. Philadelphia: J. B. Lippincott, 1980, p. 131.

BIBLIOGRAPHY

Arndt, K. A. *Manual of dermatologic therapeutics: with essentials of diagnosis,* 2nd ed. Boston: Little, Brown, 1978.

Domonkos, A. N., & Arnold, H. L. *Andrew's diseases of the skin,* 7th ed. Philadelphia: W. B. Saunders, 1982.

Fitzpatrick, T. B., et al. *Dermatology in general medicine,* 2nd ed. New York: McGraw-Hill, 1979.

Goroll, A. H., May, L. A., & Mulley, A. G. *Primary care medicine: office evaluation and management of the adult patient.* Philadelphia: J. B. Lippincott, 1981.

Hoole, A. J., Greenberg, R. A., & Pickard, C. G. *Patient care guidelines for family nurse practitioners.* Boston: Little, Brown, 1976.

Robbins, A. S., & Tamkin, J. A. *Manual of ambulatory medicine.* Philadelphia: W. B. Saunders, 1979.

CHAPTER **13**

TRAUMA

Jamie S. Brodie

Injuries and accidents constitute a significant health problem for children, resulting in death, disability, and large expenditures for their treatment and care. Accidents are the leading cause of death among children between the ages of 1 and 14 and account for 45% of deaths in this age group. Motor vehicle accidents result in 20% of all childhood deaths. In addition to motor vehicle accidents, burns, poisoning, and child abuse are common injuries in young children; older children are more prone to recreation-and play-related accidents, including falls, bicycle accidents, drownings and contact sport injuries (1).

Many childhood accidents are preventable through greater knowledge and awareness of health hazards and safety. Some states have passed child restraint laws that significantly reduce infant and child mortality from automobile accidents. The nurse practitioner can help prevent acccidental injuries to children by teaching parents to anticipate and protect their children from preventable hazards. Parents also must teach their children safety measures. The simple act of encouraging parents to properly restrain children while in an automobile can significantly reduce the risk of a fatal injury.

POISONING

The ingestion of toxic substances is common among infants and young children. The incidence of childhood poisoning has declined significantly in recent years because of public awareness of this hazard, the development of poison control centers, and the introduction of childproof caps and packaging for potentially toxic substances.

Despite a reduction in mortality from poisoning, toxic substances still result in 5% of the nonmotor vehicle-related deaths in children under 5 years of age. Of these, over half involve the ingestion or overdosage of drugs or medications (2).

PREVENTION

The goal of counseling is to prevent needless childhood poisonings. Medications should be stored in a locked cabinet out of reach of children. Toxic household products and insecticides should not be stored under the sink, but rather in a locked cabinet. Medications and many toxic household products are available in childproof packaging. Parents should not refer to medication as "candy" in order to coax a child into taking it. Children can be taught at an early age about the dangers of eating mushrooms, plants, cleaning agents, medications, etc. Parents should be provided with the telephone number of the nearest poison control center and instructed to keep it near the telephone. Teach parents first aid measures to use when a poisoning occurs.

HISTORY

Childhood poisoning often presents with an anxious phone call from the parent or babysitter. The parent may discover the child ingesting a toxic substance or find evidence suggesting poisoning, such as partially emptied containers. The parent is rarely sure about the quantity of the substance ingested and the child, fearing punishment, may either deny or be less than truthful in describing what has been ingested. Injection or inhalation of toxic substances rarely occurs in young children but may be a finding in older children or adolescents. Sometimes the child appears with a sudden onset of unusual and unexplained symptons, including drowsiness, convulsions, and vomiting. Further examination is required to rule out poisoning.

Determine, if possible, the type of toxic agent involved. The parent should be instructed to bring the container or a sample of the plant or substance, if possible. The review of system and history should be directed towards signs and symptoms associated with the toxic agent involved. The most common substances ingested by children are medications, household cleaning agents or supplies, plants, pesticides, and gardening materials.

PHYSICAL EXAMINATION

Physical findings usually are consistent with the type of substance involved, the degree of toxicity, route of consumption, amount consumed, and time delay since consumption. Particularly note any signs of central nervous system stimulation or depression, including drowsiness, unsteady gait, or unconsciousness. Signs of neurotoxic agents can include both generalized and focal seizures and muscle spasms. Changes in the respiratory or cardiac status can occur in poisonings from a number of substances and should be considered significant.

DIAGNOSTIC TESTS

A sample of the substance ingested and any emesis or material from gastric lavage should be saved for toxicologic testing. Definitive treatment in the emergency room may require general toxic substance screens of blood and urine and specific blood levels.

MANAGEMENT

The nurse practitioner will most frequently be involved in the treatment of children who have ingested substances having limited toxicity, and in the inital management of more serious poisonings before making a referral. The nurse practitioner often provides phone consultation to parents with instructions on first aid, which can significantly reduce morbidity and mortality. The local or regional poison control center is another resource that can be consulted for initial management and treatment of poisonings. Initial treatment of toxic substance ingestion is directed toward elimination of the substance from the body and limiting absorption. Vomiting should be stimulated unless corrosive substances (strong acids, alkali, or petroleum based substances) have been ingested or there is danger of aspiration due to seizures or loss of consciousness. Vomiting is safely induced in children 5 years and under by administering Syrup of Ipecac 15 cc followed by a large quantity of water. If emesis does not occur, the dose may be repeated once. Children over age 5 are administered 30 cc Syrup of Ipecac followed by water, which can be repeated once if necessary. Protect the child from aspirating vomitus by having the child bend over during emesis. If Syrup of Ipecac is unavailable, vomiting can be induced by gagging with a finger or administering a mixture of mustard and water.

Referral

Children who ingest moderately to dangerously toxic agents should be referred immediately to an emergency room for care. Consult the poison control center for specific treatment and referral recommendations.

CHILD ABUSE

Child abuse is a serious problem that results in needless suffering, injury, and death of children. It is difficult to pinpoint accurately the incidence of child abuse because many cases never reach the health care provider or are unrecognized and therefore listed as accidents.

The definition of child abuse varies for reporting purposes but includes the infliction of nonaccidental physical injury to a child by a parent or care provider. Broader definitions include neglect, emotional and sexual abuse of children. There are over 250,000 incidents of physical abuse of children reported in the United States each year. Two-thirds of these children are under 3 years of age. Recent child protection legislation has increased public awareness of child abuse and has helped bring treatment and intervention to families where it is needed (2).

HISTORY

When an abused child is brought to the clinic or emergency room for treatment of an alleged accident, frequently the explanation of circumstances surrounding the accident is vague and may be inconsistent with the extent of injury observed; for example, a child with multiple bruises and a skull fracture who is reported to have fallen out of bed. Another strong clue may be an unexplained and often inappropriate delay by the parent in seeking proper treatment for the child. In 80% of the cases, the delay is over 24 hours. This is in sharp contrast to the natural tendency of parents to seek treatment for a child soon after an accident or injury.

Take a separate history of the accident from the parent and child if possible. Note any previous history of trauma, as child abuse rarely occurs as an isolated incident. Frequently, there is a history of unexplained accidents or injuries indicative of abuse over a period of time. It is not uncommon for a child to cover up the truth about an injury in order to protect the parent.

A high incidence of child abuse exists among infants and children who were born prematurely or who experienced significant postnatal illness or failure to thrive. The mother may characterize the child as "different," physically smaller, funny looking, cries a lot, or in some way standing out from siblings in the home.

Additional clues to potential child abuse are found by taking a social and family history. Most parents who abuse children were themselves abused as children. Such parents are often socially immature and have poor adaptive and coping skills. Stress in the home is prominently associated with child abuse. Usually multiple stressors are present, including financial difficulty, recent job changes, marital discord, separation or divorce with the stress of maintaining a single parent family. A lack of parenting skills is a common finding that contributes to the neglect of the child. The parent may have unrealistic expectations of the child and may believe that strict and harsh punishment is required to make a child obey.

PHYSICAL EXAMINATION

Observe the interaction between the parent and child; this can provide clues to the degree of parental attachment. Is something "different" about this child? Is the child well nourished? Does the child appear well cared for and happy? Does the child demonstrate cognitive and motor skills appropriate to normal growth and development?

Observe the child for evidence of recent or past contusions, lacerations, bites, burns, and other injuries. Note any bruises on the head and face, or multiple bruises on the trunk, genitalia, or extremities that may be in various stages of healing. Unexplained lacerations or multiple scars should also be noted. Burns warrant close examination as cigarette burns, extensive scalds, or other patterns may be found that are inconsistent with the history provided. Palpate for areas of underlying tenderness or injury, which can include multiple fractures, sprains, and internal injuries. A complete neurologic examination is indicated since head injuries are common in cases of child abuse. An eye examination may reveal retinal hemorrhage resulting from a head injury. Fractures are sometimes manifested by a limp or a child who won't use an arm.

DIAGNOSTIC TESTS

Where there is a strong suspicion of child abuse in children under 5, roentgenographic examination may include total body x-ray films. Roentgenograms of older children may be more selective, however, they are important in the detection of recent and old fractures.

MANAGEMENT

The first priority in the management of suspected child abuse is to protect the child. Failure to intervene on behalf of the child can result in further injury or death. Ideally, the child is admitted to the hospital for additional workup, protection, and to permit investigation of the abuse. Health professionals have a legal and ethical obligation to report all suspected cases of child abuse or unexplained injury to the Child Protective Services Agency or the police. Appropriate treatment is provided to the injuries. The Protective Services Agency normally assumes responsibility for investigation and case management.

HEAD INJURIES

Head injuries represent a significant percentage of the childhood mortality and morbidity resulting from motor vehicle accidents, child abuse, falls, bicycle accidents, contact sports, and other recreational injuries. Although serious injuries to the head are generally referred to an emergency room physician for care, the nurse practitioner may be involved in the treatment of children with minor head injuries, including closed head injuries not associated with unconsciousness and minor scalp contusions and lacerations. It is essential that the nurse practitioner carefully evaluate the child with a head injury by means of a detailed history, physical examination, and observation, when necessary, to rule out a more serious injury.

HISTORY

Typically, the child appears with a recent blow to the head accompanied by pain, dizziness, "seeing stars," or temporary disorientation. Any report of unconsciousness following the injury should be reported to a physician for care. It is important to note the approximate time of the injury, and the presence of any subsequent symptoms, including nausea, vomiting, headache, drowsiness, seizures, amnesia, or nervousness.

PHYSICAL EXAMINATION

Carefully inspect and palpate the head and scalp for contusions, lacerations, or irregularities. A neurologic examination should be conducted to include observation of appearance and behavior, mental status, gait, cranial nerves, tendon reflexes, and motor function. Vital signs should be recorded, and the child observed for signs of increased intracranial pressure.

DIAGNOSTIC TESTS

X-ray skull films may be ordered when the injury is associated with unconsciousness, when a skull fracture is suspected, or when the neurologic examination demonstrates evidence of pathology. The treatment of a minor head injury focuses on the relief of discomfort, and observation to rule out more serious injury.

MANAGEMENT

Minor head injuries can be managed safely by the nurse practitioner on an outpatient basis if arrangements can be made for observation of the child for possible sequelae of the injury. Usually, the parent or a family member can be enlisted for this purpose. Typically, the child will experience soreness or minor discomfort at the site of the injury, a headache, giddiness, or fatigue. In rare cases, a child with no history of unconsciousness or signs of significant injury at the time of examination may subsequently develop signs of a concussion, traumatic brain edema, epidural hemorrhage, or subdural hematoma. The onset of neurologic symptoms can occur hours, days, or weeks after a seemingly minor injury.

After a head injury, only minor analgesics, such as aspirin or acetaminophen (Tylenol) in therapeutic dosages should be used. Analgesics that have the potential to alter the level of consciousness or mask significant neurologic changes are not used. Ice packs may be applied to scalp contusions to decrease the swelling and pain.

Counseling

The parent should be advised to immediately report any seizures, weakness, increased headaches, persistent or projectile vomiting, unconsciousness or stupor, unequal pupils, confusion, or behavioral changes. For the first night after the injury, the child should be awakened periodically throughout the night to detect any developing neurologic signs or symptoms.

Referral

The development of significant neurologic signs, evidence of increased intracranial pressure, or signs of major head trauma necessitate immediate referral to a physician for care.

BURNS

In the United States, burns are the second leading cause of death in children younger than 5 years of age, and the third leading cause of death in children between ages 5 and 14. The majority of burns in children occur in the home, usually in the kitchen or bathroom. Burns can result from contact with flames, hot objects, hot liquids, chemical exposure, radiation, electrical current, or extreme cold; however, scalds are the most common burn injury among infants and children less than 5 years old. Older children are most frequently burned by open flames ignited from flammable clothing. While extensive or severe burns are necessarily referred for physician or hospital care, the nurse practitioner frequently will encounter minor burns that can safely and easily be managed on an outpatient basis (3).

THERMAL BURNS

History

Note the source of the burn, any concurrent trauma, whether chemical or electrical agents were involved, the date of the last tetanus booster, and the amount of time elapsed since the burn occurred. It is important to inquire about any respiratory involvement, including shortness of breath, smoke inhalation, soot in the mouth, or facial burns. The presence of a chronic illness, such as diabetes, or cardiac illness will affect the clinical course and management of the burn and should be noted. The age of the child is an important consideration since infants and young children are more prone to complications, including disorders of fluid balance, heat loss, increased caloric requirements, and respiratory complications.

Physical Examination

There are three factors that must be considered when evaluating burns: (1) the location of the burn; (2) the depth or degree of tissue damage; and (3) the extent of body surface involvement. The location of a burn is significant because some areas of the body present unusual management problems, risk of complications, or increased potential for disability. Serious burns involving the face, hands, feet, or genitals should be referred immediately for physician care.

Burns are evaluated as to the depth of tissue damage and classified according to degree. Determining the depth of tissue damage may not always be possible at the time of initial examination and may have to wait until further signs of damage become apparent.

First degree burns are superficial, partial-thickness burns involving the epidermis, and commonly result from excessive exposure to the sun or a heat contact of short duration. First degree burns usually cause pain, mild hyperesthesia, and erythema. The skin remains dry and sensitive to pressure, touch, and temperature, with blistering or edema minimal or absent.

Second degree burns are partial-thickness burns involving the epidermis and the dermis layers of the skin. They usually result from scalds or brief contact with a heat source, and cause pain, hyperesthesia, sensitivity to touch and temperature, and a moist, blistered or weeping surface.

Third degree burns are a full thickness burn involving destruction of the epidermis and dermis layers with damage to the subcutaneous tissue. They result from direct contact with a flame or heat source, and have a dry leathery appearance which can be white or charred. The burn is usually not painful or sensitive to touch or pressure because of destruction to the pain receptors. Third degree burns are always referred to a physician for care since proper healing requires surgical treatment and specialized care.

Management

First degree burns usually heal rapidly with few complications. Treatment is largely directed toward making the client comfortable and can include application of ice packs, cold soaks, soothing creams, topical anesthetic agents, and analgesia. Typically, the area will peel seven to ten days after the burn.

Second degree burns can be managed by the nurse practitioner when:

1. The extent of the burn is limited
2. No chronic illness exists that could influence the course of the burn treatment
3. There is no significant involvement of the face, hands, feet, or genitalia, and no circumferential burns
4. The client is not an infant

When determining the extent of a burn, it may be helpful to consult a reference containing the *Rule of Nines* or similar chart for measurement of percent of body surface. The goals in treating second degree burns are to prevent infection, promote healing through adequate wound care, and promote comfort.

Initial management of a second degree burn includes ice water soaks for comfort, and cleansing of the burned area with a mild detergent and tap water or sterile saline. Do not rupture blisters that remain intact, however, do debride loose tissue and debris. Administer tetanus prophylaxis as appropriate. Apply a petrolatum gauze and bulk Kerlix dressing. Analgesics will be necessary for relief of pain after the burn.

Healing will normally take approximately two weeks and requires followup. Depending on the motivation and ability of the parents, instruction may be provided for home care, or the child can return for daily dressing changes. Follow-up care includes soaking off of the old dressing, observation of tissue for signs of infection, and redressing of wound. Topical or systemic antibiotics may be used for infection occurring during treatment.

Counseling. Counseling is directed toward burn prevention. Many burns are preventable through greater knowledge and awareness of fire hazards, precautions to be taken around open flames, and planned emergency fire procedures. Sunburns in children can be largely prevented by using readily available sunscreens and by limiting exposure time. Parents should be encouraged to buy flame-retardant pajamas and other clothing for their children, and children should be taught the proper safety procedure to follow in the event of clothing ignition. Parents of infants and young children need counseling about the danger of scald injuries and should be instructed to test the temperature of bath water with their wrist before bathing a child.

Pharmacology. Drug treatment of the child with a burn injury includes the provision of tetanus prophylaxis as needed, analgesics, and topical or systemic antibiotics as required to prevent or control infection. Aspirin or acetaminophen (Tylenol) in dosages appropriate to the child's age and weight is recommended for relief of pain for a minor burn. More extensive burns may require intermediate range analgesics or narcotic analgesics. Topical antibiotics and antiinfectives, including silver sulfadiazine cream, can be applied for the prevention or treatment of localized infection. Oral antibiotics can be used for extensive infection, cellulitis associated with a burn injury, or prophylaxis where a dirty wound exists.

ELECTRICAL BURNS

Electrical burns are caused by the passage of an electrical current through portions of the body, resulting in tissue damage. In children, electrical burns most often result from a child chewing on an electrical cord. In addition to tissue destruction, electrical current can produce cardiac arrhythmias and cardiorespiratory arrest. Normally, an electrical burn will result in entry and exit wound through which the current has passed. Often, the tissue and organ damage is not visible and may be disproportionately large in comparison to the size of the entry-exit wounds. It is for this reason that children with electrical burns are referred to a physician for care.

CHEMICAL BURNS

Chemical burns result from exposure to a corrosive acid or alkali substance that produces tissue damage or destruction. Depending on the agent and the duration of exposure, a chemical burn can be either partial or full thickness.

The immediate treatment is to flush the surface with copious amounts of water to remove the chemical and prevent its penetration to deeper tissues. After removal of the chemical agent, the burn can be treated in the same manner as a thermal burn, according to the extent, depth, and location of tissue damage.

EYE TRAUMA

The nurse practitioner is often required to evaluate and treat eye injuries. Over two million eye injuries occur each year in the United States. They are commonly the result of blunt trauma to the eye, foreign bodies, and chemical burns.

Many eye injuries can be prevented through greater use of protective devices for the eye. Safety goggles are particularly important when working with power saws, grinders, mowers, hammers, and chisels, or around corrosive chemicals. Children involved in contact sports should be counseled about the importance of wearing face shields and helmets for protection.

In all cases of eye injury a detailed history should be taken as to the circumstances surrounding the injury. Get a description of the object involved in blunt trauma, or the suspected composition of a foreign body or chemical agent. Typically, the child with eye trauma or a foreign body will have pain, redness, photophobia, excessive tearing, diplopia, blurred vision, or change in visual status. Always inquire about the visual status in both eyes before the injury occurred, and note any previous history of eye trauma, disease, and whether corrective lenses are usually worn.

With the exception of chemical burns, it is crucial that the visual acuity be measured in both eyes before examination or treatment; this serves as a baseline against which subsequent improvement or deterioration can be measured. All cases of eye injury should be followed up in 24 hours. When an eye injury or foreign body is associated with pain, examination can be facilitated by use of a topical anesthetic. Tetracaine hydrochloride 1% (Pontocaine) may be instilled to promote comfort during examination, but should never be prescribed for self administration by the client at home.

CHEMICAL BURNS

Treatment should be immediate and should consist of eye irrigation with tap water or sterile normal saline solution. Eye irrigation should be continued for *20 to 30 minutes* to flush the agent from the eye and conjunctival folds. In general, alkaline burns are more damaging than acid burns. Minor chemical burns can be treated with irrigation only, or in combination with analgesics and an ophthalmic antibiotic. After irrigation, an examination is performed, including testing of visual acuity, examination of the conjunctiva, cornea, and fundus. After a minor chemical irritation, the cornea is typically clear and the conjunctiva is pink, vascular, or sometimes hemorrahgic. Immediately refer to an ophthalmologist any child with a hazy or opaque cornea, corneal erosion, or a white, avascular conjunctiva.

BLUNT TRAUMA

Examination of the child with blunt trauma to the eye should include testing for visual acuity, palpation of the orbital margins and nasal bridge, examination of extraocular motions, examination of the lids, adnexa, conjunctiva, and pupils, and funduscopic examination. Blunt trauma to the eye can produce the following conditions, which should be ruled out: (*1*) hyphema; (*2*) corneal lacerations; (*3*) retinal detachment; and (*4*) orbital fractures.

Periorbital edema and ecchymosis (black eye) are common childhood conditions that result from blunt trauma, and can be treated with cold compresses and an analgesic. Unless massive, subconjunctival hemorrhages are usually benign and will clear up without treatment. Any signs of visual disturbance, excessive pain, or suspicion of the aforementioned conditions should be referred to an ophthalmologist for evaluation and care.

FOREIGN BODY

Foreign bodies in the eye can range from specks of dust, which are easily removed, to penetrating objects which, require removal by an ophthalmologist. Typically, a child will have a history of a foreign body in the eye and complain of redness, pain, and tearing. Note the composition of the foreign body, for example, sand, metal, or wood, and the activity that resulted in injury. Examination should include visual acuity testing and full ophthalmic examination. Pontocaine 1% may be administered before examination if significant pain is present. During examination, the upper and lower eyelids are everted and any foreign bodies removed using a sterile applicator moistened with sterile saline solution. Visualizations of small foreign bodies is aided through the use of an oblique, moving bright illumination, such as the slit setting on an ophthalmoscope or a slit lamp. Foreign bodies embedded in the cornea will require removal by an ophthalmologist.

Often, examination will reveal no foreign body, however, there may be corneal abrasions. Corneal injuries produce intense pain. Fluorescein 1 or 2% is an indicator dye used to detect abrasions or defects in the surface of the cornea. The eye is first anesthetized with Pontocaine 1% and the fluorescein is applied. Fluorescein is commonly available on sterile paper strips that are impregnated with the dye. The strip is touched to the lower conjunctival sac near the inner canthus where tears dissolve the fluorescein and spread it across the surface of the eye. An abrasion or break in the surface of the cornea permits the penetration and accumulation of the dye. The eye is irrigated with sterile saline or Dacriose solution. Any abrasions or breaks will retain the dye, and then can be easily identified. A blue or black light is sometimes used to intensify the color of the dye retaining defects.

Superficial corneal abrasions require careful management, because a break in the corneal epithelium increases the risk of infection and the potential for corneal scars if not properly treated. An antibiotic ointment is applied (sulfacetamide or neomycin sulfate [Neosporin Ophthalmic]) and the eye patched for 24 hours, after which the eye is reexamined. Healing normally requires 24 hours and rarely 48 hours, and is evidenced by a lack of pain and the failure to stain with fluorescein. Always document visual acuity on a follow-up visit.

Referral

The nurse practitioner should only treat superficial eye injuries at low risk of complications. Clients with serious chemical burns, lacerations, embedded foreign bodies, or evidence of intraocular damage should be referred to an ophthalmologist for care.

LACERATIONS AND ABRASIONS

Nurse practitioners, particularly those in rural areas, frequently see children with minor abrasions and lacerations that are easily managed in the outpatient setting. The following is a review of the assessment, management, and follow-up of lacerations and is not designed as a definitive text on skin closure. It is recommended that nurse practitioners consult textbooks on wound healing, wound evaluation, and skin closure and receive clinical instruction before undertaking skin closure with sutures.

In general, the nurse practitioner will treat only superficial lacerations not involving the face or having other cosmetic implications. Facial wounds, lacerations involving significant underlying tissue damage, and wounds requiring complex closure or where significant tissue loss or infection has occurred will be referred to a physician for care. Wounds over six hours old are at higher risk for subsequent infection clients with such wounds should also be referred to a physician.

When evaluating abrasions, contusions, or lacerations, it is important to take an accurate history of the circumstances surrounding the injury, including the time of the injury. A complete history can provide information on the likelihood of subsequent infection and the presence of foreign bodies in the wound. Always inquire about the date of the client's last immunization for tetanus. Examine the wound, noting its size, depth, presence of foreign bodies, and involvement of underlying structures. On the hand or extremities, check for damages to the tendons or underlying muscles by having the child demonstrate the full range of motion or function of the hand or limb. A slight paresthesia is normal for the skin adjacent to the laceration; however, in extensive or deep lacerations it is important to check for nerve damage. Any evidence of arterial bleeding should be controlled with pressure the client and referred to a physician.

ABRASIONS

Abrasions involve damage to the outer layers of skin, usually through a scrape against a rough surface. Although superficial, abrasions can easily become infected by contamination from dirt, road gravel, and other agents. Bleeding is usually slight; however, the wound may ooze. Management includes tetanus prophylaxis if necessary and vigorous cleansing of the abrasion with Betadine Scrub or similar antiseptic cleanser. Sometimes it is helpful to use a small scrub brush when dirt is embedded. Apply an antibiotic ointment (Neosporin or Betadine); healing usually occurs rapidly. The parents should be advised to report any signs of infection.

LACERATIONS

Bleeding can usually be controlled with direct pressure. Before repair, the wound is cleaned with Betadine Scrub or an antiseptic soap and water. Any obvious foreign bodies are gently removed, and the skin surrounding the wound is shaved. The wound is irrigated with saline solution. Determine the involvement of underlying tendons, muscles, nerves, arteries, and other structures. If it appears that damage to these has occurred, it will be necessary to refer the child to a physician for care. Superficial lacerations often can be closed with Steri-Strips or butterfly skin closures, with satisfactory healing occurring in five to eight days. A small pressure dressing may be applied for hemostasis, and tetanus prophylaxis is administered as appropriate.

More extensive lacerations will require closure with sutures. Young children usually require restraint before repair of a laceration. The placement of sutures is always done with sterile technique, using sterile instruments, gloves, solutions, drapes, suture, gauze, and other supplies. The primary goal is to produce a skin closure with accurate tissue approximation and to promote healing in a manner that is both cosmetic and free from infection.

After cleaning the wound and shaving the surrounding area, the wound is draped with sterile drapes and painted with Betadine solution. Anesthetize the wound by infiltrating the surrounding tissue with 1% Xylocaine, using a 26-gauge needle. The wound is again irrigated with sterile saline solution and further evaluation is made of the depth and extent of damage to the underlying structures. The wound is probed for foreign bodies and debrided as necessary to provide a smooth closure. A scalpel or tissue scissors are used to trim macerated or irregular tissue surfaces in order to produce a smooth closure that will heal rapidly. Often it is necessary to incise the entire laceration, as rough, jagged edges can delay healing and increase scar formation.

A general principle of simple wound closure is to approximate like tissue in a manner that will minimize tension on the outer layer of skin. Close approximation of the outer layers with minimal tension will result in a more cosmetic closure. The two primary means of reducing tension on the surface of the wound are to close underlying layers with retention sutures and to undermine the surface layer of skin.

Selection of Sutures

A variety of suture material is commercially available, and in general, these are categorized as either absorbable or nonabsorbable. Absorbable suture is manufactured from sheep intestine and is referred to as plain, chromic, or gut suture. It is used for internal sutures that will be left to dissolve and be absorbed.

Nonabsorbable sutures are used for the external closure of the wound and must be removed after healing is sufficient to maintain skin integrity. Nonabsorbable sutures are manufactured from a number of natural and synthetic agents, including silk, nylon, and prolene, and can be monofilament or braided.

Suture Sizes

Suture size and strength range from 1-0 (pronounced one-oh), which is maximum strength, through 6-0, which is extremely delicate and is used for fine cosmetic work. Clinically, suture is selected to match the strength of the tissue being sutured and the degree of tension that will be placed on it. Typically, a minor laceration without cosmetic implications can be closed with a 3-0 plain absorbable retention sutures and 4-0 nylon sutures for external closure.

The laceration is closed in layers to prevent tissue gaps which increase the likelihood of a wound infection and promote scar formation. The best results are obtained by using interrupted sutures tied with a square knot. Because knots easily become loosened, at least 3 to 4 knots should be tied.

Sutures should be removed when healing has occurred sufficiently to maintain skin integrity. Seven to nine days is adequate for most wounds; however, where cosmetic results are desired, as in facial wounds, sutures will be removed in five to six days. In general, the longer the suture remains in place, the greater is the likelihood of a localized reaction to the suture material.

Counseling

The parents should be instructed to observe the suture site carefully for signs of infection, such as redness, swelling, bleeding, breaking open, or draining pus. Instruction concerning wound care should include when and how to replace dry dressings, the importance of keeping the suture site dry, and when to return for suture removal or follow-up care.

SPRAINS

Traumatic injuries to the knee and ankle are common among school-age children and children involved in contact sports. Careful examination and assessment permits the nurse practitioner to gauge the extent of damage and provide appropriate treatment for minor to moderate sprains.

A sprain involves the partial tearing of a ligament and joint capsule, resulting in pain, swelling, and joint laxity. A sprain can be minor with only mild tearing of the ligamentous fibers or moderate to severe with more extensive damage. The complete tearing of a ligament is referred to as a ruptured ligament.

ANKLE SPRAIN

Ankle sprains most frequently involve the lateral ligaments, producing pain and swelling on the lateral side of the ankle. These sprains commonly result from a forced inversion of the ankle, usually while the foot is in plantar flexion. The lateral supporting ligaments of the ankle are: (*1*) the anterior talofibular ligament, (*2*) the calcaneofibular ligament, and (*3*) the posterior talofibular ligament. The medial supporting ligament is the deltoid ligament, which is less commonly injured.

History

The child may have a recent history of "twisting the ankle" or a fall, with the immediate or subsequent onset of pain, swelling, difficulty walking, or joint instability. He or she may report having walked after the injury with the later development of acute pain. It is important to note the cause and mechanism of the injury or stress applied to the ankle.

Physical Examination

The physical examination should progress in an orderly manner and include direct observation. Note any swelling, ecchymosis, or obvious deformity. Throughout the examination, comparisons should be made to the noninjured ankle. Gently palpate the ankle, noting point tenderness over the medial and lateral tendons. Evaluate the circulatory status of the foot and ankle and assess the range of motion. Any abnormal range of motion is indicative of a ruptured ligament. Perform an *anterior drawer test* of the ankle by grasping the lower leg with one hand and pulling the heel anteriorly with the other. A positive drawer sign is indicative of a ruptured anterior talofibular ligament, which will require further evaluation and treatment by an orthopedist.

Diagnostic Tests

In all but the most minor sprains, it will be necessary to obtain x-ray films. Anterior-posterior (AP) lateral, and oblique films are necessary to rule out fractures and avulsion fractures.

Management

Minor ankle sprains are easily managed with crutches, elevation, ice packs, an Ace wrap, and analgesics for pain. A useful ice pack can be made from a plastic garbage bag filled with ice, which easily molds to the shape of the extremity. Hot packs can be used for comfort 24 to 48 hours after injury. As swelling and pain decreases, ambulation can be started as tolerated. Range of motion exercises are useful and an Ace wrap can be maintained to provide support to the ankle.

Unfortunately, ligaments are not highly vascular and as a result tend to heal slowly. Complete healing of a ligament injury can take one to three months or more. During this period, the ankle joint is somewhat unstable and easily prone to reinjury.

Counseling.   Parents and child must be counseled on the etiology of the sprain and the necessity of avoiding activities or sports likely to reinjure the ankle for a period of a month to six weeks, or until full healing and ankle stability occur. The parents should be taught how to care for the ankle during the recovery period; the health care provider should initially stress the need for application of ice packs and elevation of the ankle, and should tell the parents how to reapply the Ace wrap for comfort and support. The parents should be advised to return the child for follow-up care and to report any "giving away" of the ankle, ankle instability, pain, or swelling that persists.

Referral.   The nurse practitioner should refer to an orthopedist any child who has a severe sprain characterized by joint instability, evidence of a ruptured ligament, severe lateral and medial swelling, evidence of ankle fracture, or obvious deformity to an orthopedist.

KNEE SPRAINS

The nurse practitioner often must evaluate and treat minor knee injuries. The most prevalent injuries to the knee involve:

1. Ligamentous injuries
2. Injury or tears of the meniscus
3. Patellar injuries or damage to the extensor mechanism of the knee

Children with patellar and meniscal injuries are always referred to an orthopedist; however, it is important that the nurse practitioner be able to evaluate and treat minor ligamentous injuries or sprains of the knee.

History

In children, knee injuries often result from falls or torsional stress on the knee, which can occur in sports and other activities. Inquire about the mechanism of injury and direction in which the knee was stressed. Note the onset of symptoms and any previous history of knee injury or "trick knee." Also note whether symptoms were gradual in onset or occurred immediately after the injury and whether the child was able to walk after the injury. Tears of the miniscus are often accompanied by pain, swelling, and limitation in range of motion, which develops over a period of time. Because meniscal injuries can mimic other knee disorders, any stable knee disorder that fails to improve within a reasonable period of time should be referred for additional evaluation.

Physical Examination

It is desirable to examine the knee as soon after an injury as possible before swelling, pain, and effusion make the examination more difficult. Keep in mind that muscle guarding, pain, or effusion can make examination difficult and mask important signs and symptoms. Begin the examination by inspecting both knees, using the noninjured knee for comparison. Note any deformity of the knee or misplacement of the patella, which can be indicative of a dislocation or other serious injury. Note the presence of swelling, effusion, or ecchymosis. Gently palpate the knee noting point of maximum tenderness. Tenderness over the patella may indicate a patellar fracture. Note the range of motion of both knees and any difficulty fully extending the knee.

Check the ability of the child to extend the knee against force or do leg lifts with the legs in extension. The inability to perform this maneuver can indicate serious injury to the extensor mechanism, including a displaced patellar fracture, rupture of a patellar ligament, rupture of the quadriceps insertion; it also can be symptomatic of a torn meniscus.

Check for instability of the knee by applying firm stress from both the lateral and medial surfaces of the knee with the knee in the flexed and extended positions. Also perform an anterior and posterior drawer test for instability in that plane. If abnormal joint motion can be detected in either plane, a ruptured ligament is suspected and must be referred.

Diagnostic Tests

With the exception of minor knee sprains, roentgenographic examination of the knee is necessary and should include AP and lateral views to rule out fractures and avulsion injuries.

Management

Minor knee sprains that are stable can easily be managed by the nurse practitioner. Initial treatment includes ice packs, elevation of knee, ace wrap or knee support, analgesics, and crutches if the child is unable to ambulate. As pain and swelling diminish, ambulation and isometric quadricep exercises are helpful in restoring stability and reducing joint laxity.

Counseling.   The parents should be instructed on proper care of the knee, stressing the need for application of ice and elevation of the knee during the initial period of swelling and pain. As swelling diminishes, the child may begin quadriceps exercises and initiate ambulation, using caution to avoid activities likely to reinjure the knee. The parents and child should be instructed to report any "giving away" of the knee or persistent pain or swelling. Teach the child to perform isometric quadricep exercises: 15 to 20 contractions repeated five to eight times per day.

Referral.   With the exception of minor knee sprains, the majority of knee injuries are appropriately referred to an orthopedist for consultation, evaluation, or care. Moderate knee sprains often are treated initially by the nurse practitioner, with an orthopedic consultation following in several days. Always refer children who show signs of fractures, extensor mechanism injuries, ruptured ligaments, joint instability, a locked knee, or a child with persistent pain or swelling.

STUDY QUESTIONS

Circle all that apply.

1. In the United States, the leading cuase of accidental deaths in children is:

   a. burns
   b. falls
   c. drowning
   d. motor vehicle accidents

2. The nurse practitioner receives a telephone call from a mother whose child, Jenny, age 2, has just eaten an entire bottle of baby aspirin that had been left open on the counter. The best initial advice would be:

   a. dilute the stomach contents by having her drink a large quantity of water
   b. bring the child to the clinic immediately for care
   c. decrease absorption by having her drink a glass of vegetable oil
   d. induce vomiting

3. Which of the following measures can help prevent childhood poisoning?

   a. store toxic substances and medications in locked storage cabinets
   b. purchase medications and hazardous products in childproof containers
   c. teach young children about the danger of eating or drinking household preparations, medications, or unknown substances
   d. keep the phone number of the poison control center near the telephone

4. The majority of child abuse cases reported in the United States involves children:

   a. less than 1 year of age
   b. less than 3 years of age
   c. 3 to 5 years of age
   d. 5 to 9 years of age

5. The health history can provide valuable clues to the identification of child abuse. Which of the following are commonly associated with child abuse?

   a. delay in seeking treatment for the child
   b. circumstances surrounding the injury are vague
   c. history is inconsistent with the extent of injury observed
   d. history of prior unexplained accident or injury
   e. child was a premature infant or is in some way "different"

6. John, age 6, fell off his bicycle today and sustained a closed head injury. He was not knocked out and his physical examination was normal. Management of this injury would include:

   a. aspirin or acetaminophen (Tylenol) for headache
   b. ice packs for contusion of scalp
   c. parents to awaken him periodically throughout the night to detect any development of neurological symptoms
   d. instruct parents to observe him for persistent vomiting, unusual change in consciousness, unequal pupils, convulsions, or a behavioral change

7. Which of the following are appropriate in the initial management of a child with a second degree burn to the anterior forearm?

   a. soak burned area in iced aline for comfort
   b. clean with mild detergent
   c. carefully rupture blisters and express liquid
   d. check date of last tetanus immunization

8. Chemical burns to the eyes are initially treated with a continuous eye irrigation for 20 to 30 minutes followed by an examination. Which of the following physical findings would require an immediate referral to an ophthalmologist?

   a. white avascular conjunctiva
   b. pink, vascular, or slightly hemorrhagic conjunctiva
   c. hazy or opaque cornea
   d. mild corneal erosion

9. A general principle of simple wound closure that can promote rapid and cosmetic healing is:

   a. close approximation of skin surface using absorbable suture
   c. close approximation of underlying tissue layers with slight overlap of surface layers
   c. close approximation of tissue layers with firm tension on skin surface
   d. close approximation of all tissue layers with minimal tension on skin surface

10. Charles, age 10, is seen in the clinic complaining of a "twisted ankle," which he sustained while playing basketball. The ankle is moderately swollen and he has a noticeable limp. On physical examination, which of the following would be consistent with a minor sprain?

   a. moderate swelling and point tenderness over the lateral ligaments of the ankle
   b. a positive anterior drawer test
   c. full range of motion with no abnormal joint movement
   d. palpable defect in the tendo calcaneous

ANSWERS

1. d	6. a, b, c, d
2. d	7. a, b, d
3. a, b, c, d	8. a, c, d
4. b	9. d
5. a, b, c, d, e	10. a, c

REFERENCES

1. U. S. Department of Health, Education and Welfare, *Health People*. Washington, D.C.: U. S. Government Printing Office, 1979.
2. Kempe, C. H., & Helfer, R. E. *The battered child*. Chicago: The University of Chicago Press, 1981.
3. Feller, I., et al., *Emergency care of the burn victim*. Ann Arbor, MI: The National Institute for Burn Medicine, 1977.

BIBLIOGRAPHY

Condon, R. E., & Nyhus, L. M. *Manual of surgical therapeutics*. Boston: Little, Brown, 1978, 457.

Feller, I., et al., *Emergency care of the burn victim*. Ann Arbor, MI: The National Institute for Burn Medicine, 1977.

Freeman, H. MacKenzie, M.D., (ED.): *Ocular trauma*. New York: Appleton-Century-Crofts, 1976.

Iverson, L. D., & Clawson, D. K. *Manual of acute orthopedics*. Boston: Little, Brown, 1977.

Kempe, C. H., & Helfer, R. E. *The battered child*. Chicago: The University of Chicago Press, 1981.

Odom, G. L. *Central nervous system trauma research status report*. Washington, D.C.: National Institute of Health, 1979.

Runyon, J. W. *Primary care guide*. New York: Harper & Row, 1975.

U. S. Department of Health, Education and Welfare, *Healthy people*. Washington, D.C.: U. S. Government Printing Office, 1979.

Wagner, M. M. *Care of the burn injured patient*. Littleton, MA: PSG Publishing, 1981.

CHAPTER 14

INFECTIOUS DISEASES

Terry E. Tippett Neilson

Before the advent of immunizations, childhood infectious diseases were very common in the American household. Although some produced only a mild illness (e.g., chickenpox and roseola), others were responsible for serious complications and even death. Currently, there are effective vaccinations for polio, rubella, measles, pertussis, and mumps. It is only where immunization practices are relaxed that localized outbreaks of these diseases occur. This chapter will discuss only those infectious diseases that involve a rash.

When assessing infectious diseases, diagnostic tests are often unnecessary. A reliable diagnosis can be based on a careful clinical history and physical examination. A complete history of the rash is the single most valuable piece of information that can be obtained. The following six questions are helpful in the differential diagnosis of an infectious disease rash:

1. Where did the rash begin and what did it look like?
2. Were there any symptoms before the rash?
3. How long did the symptoms exist before the rash?
4. Is there a history of exposure to other people with a similar rash?
5. Is the child on any medication?
6. Which immunizations has the child had?

With the exception of scarlet fever, the infectious diseases that are discussed in this chapter are viral, self-limiting illnesses. The management is symptomatic and can be easily managed by a nurse practitioner. However, if complications such as pneumonia, encephalitis, seizures, or secondary bacterial infections should develop, a physician referral and/or consultation become essential. The immunocompromised client requires physician supervision and will not be discussed in this chapter.

CHICKENPOX (VARICELLA)

Chickenpox, along with measles, is one of the most contagious viral diseases known to mankind. However, chickenpox has a far lower morbidity and mortality rate.

If the mother has a history of chickenpox, her newborn is generally protected passively for three to six months. Usually, the illness is mild and is seen most frequently in children from 2 to 8 years of age. It is spread by direct exposure with an infected person. The virus is shed from the skin vesicles (before crusting occurs) and the respiratory tract. The child is contagious from about two days before the rash appears until all lesions are crusted over. The incubation period lasts 10 to 21 days.

HISTORY AND PHYSICAL EXAMINATION

A history of mild headache, low-grade fever, malaise, anorexia, and occasionally sore throat may occur 24 to 36 hours before the rash appears. These symptoms are usually more severe in a child over the age of 10 and may be absent in very young children. Generally, the rash starts on the trunk and spreads outward. In the mild forms of the disease, the extremities and the face may be spared. If the mucous membranes are involved, the vesicles often ulcerate. The rash is maculopapular, rapidly changing to vesicles followed by crusting. Since the rash occurs in successive crops, it can be seen in all stages of development simultaneously. Secondary bacterial infections may occur from scratching the primary lesions. The duration of all the skin lesions is about 10 days.

MANAGEMENT

Since chickenpox is usually a self-limiting disease, symptomatic treatment is all that is required. To avoid secondary bacterial infections, the care giver should be instructed to clip the nails short and bathe the child frequently. Antihistamines and topical calamine lotion are useful to reduce the itching. If secondary infections occur, topical antibiotics are used. For the child with ulcerated mouth lesions, a mild soft diet is recommended. Since the use of aspirin with children who have varicella has been associated with Reye's syndrome, it is recommended that acetaminophen is used to control fever.

GERMAN MEASLES (RUBELLA)

German measles is not as contagious as chickenpox or measles. Before the advent of the rubella immunization, many children would escape the illness and get it as young adults. It is a very mild disease, rarely causing any complications. The fetus, however, can suffer severe malformations and/or widely disseminated disease if the mother contracts the illness during the first trimester of her pregnancy.

The rubella virus is shed from the nasopharyngeal tract as well as the urine, stool, and blood; therefore, the disease can be spread by direct contact with an infected person or by freshly contaminated articles. The person is contagious from seven days before the rash until five days after the appearance of the rash. The incubation period is between 14 to 21 days. One attack of rubella generally renders a permanent immunity, however, prevention through vaccination is the best path to follow.

HISTORY AND PHYSICAL EXAMINATION

Before the rash develops, the prodromal signs and symptoms are either very mild or absent. A history of mild fever, headache, malaise, sore throat, coryza may be reported. Enlarged posterior auricular, posterior cervical, and occipital lymph nodes with a rash is pathognomonic for rubella.

The rose-colored maculopapular rash begins on the face and proceeds down the body in a linear fashion. After about 36 hours, the rash will reach the feet and begin to fade in a similar sequence. About the second or third day of the rash, some people experience mild arthritis in several joints. This is more common with young adults and lasts about two to three weeks.

MANAGEMENT

The care is symptomatic. Aspirin for the mild fever, headache, and arthritic-like symptoms is often prescribed. The client and/or care giver must be educated to avoid pregnant women and large crowded areas for five days after the appearance of the rash.

ROSEOLA INFANTUM (EXANTHEMA SUBITUM)

Little is known about this common disease of early childhood. It is believed to be caused by a virus, however, the mode of transmission, period of communicability, and incubation period are not firmly established. Roseola is frequently seen in very young children between the ages of 3 months to 3 years. During the spring and fall, localized outbreaks are common.

HISTORY AND PHYSICAL EXAMINATION

To an unsuspecting mother, roseola can be a frightening disease. There is a sudden onset of very high fever (104° to 106° F is not uncommon) in a previously well child. Occasionally accompanying the fever, there may be a mild cough and red throat. With the exception of enlarged occipital lymph nodes, the physical examination is unremarkable. After three to four days, the fever disappears as abruptly as it arrived and there is the onset of the rash.

The rash of roseola is nonpruritic, pink-red maculopapular. Usually it is more diffused on the trunk and neck and spare on the face and extremities. The duration of the rash is between one to three days.

MANAGEMENT

Frequently, the diagnosis of this illness is not made until the fever falls and rash appears. The three to four days of high fever can be very unsettling for both the mother and the nurse practitioner. Management is symptomatic. Aspirin or acetaminophen, and tepid baths are used to control the fever. To prevent dehydration, adequate fluid intake is essential.

MEASLES (RUBEOLA)

Measles is a highly contagious disease. Before the rubeola vaccination, it was estimated that 98% of the population had measles. Since immunization is so effective, measles is becoming a very rare disease. It is only where immunization practices are relaxed that localized outbreaks occur. If the mother has either had measles or has been vaccinated against measles, the newborn is believed to be passively protected up to 15 months of age. Therefore, immunization with the live attenuated measle virus should not be administered until the child is 15 months old, the only exception being when there is a localized outbreak of measles in the community. However, the child will need to be revaccinated at the age of 15 months if vaccinated before 13 months.

Rubeola is spread by respiratory tract secretions. The incubation period is between 9 to 14 days. The child is contagious from the fifth day of the incubation period to the fifth or sixth day of the rash.

Unlike the other infectious diseases discussed in this chapter, measles has a significantly higher incidence of morbidity and mortality. Some of the complications of this disease are otitis media, pneumonia, and encephalitis.

HISTORY AND PHYSICAL EXAMINATION

Measles generally begins with a fever of 103° to 104° F and malaise. Within 24 hours after the fever, coryza, conjunctivitis, and cough occur. The rash usually appears about four days after the onset of the illness. Koplik's spots are pathognomonic for measles. These are red eruptions with white spots in the center, located on the buccal mucosa opposite the first and second molars. They occur 24 to 36 hours before the rash and disappear approximately 24 hours after the appearance of the rash.

The rash begins at the back of the neck, around the ears, and the hairline. It proceeds down the body in a linear pattern. After about five days it will usually reach the feet and begin to fade in the same sequence, the duration being about 10 days. The rash is described as dark pink-purple maculopapular lesions.

MANAGEMENT

Since this is a highly contagious disease, the infected child should be isolated from the onset of the illness until the fifth day of the rash. As with all viral illnesses, symptomatic care is all that can be offered. The mother should be instructed to keep the child in bed until the child is afebrile for two to three days. No special diet is required, however, adequate fluid intake is essential to prevent dehydration. Aspirin or acetaminophen may be used to control the fever. Since the child is often photophobic, bright lights should be avoided.

SCARLET FEVER (SCARLATINA)

Scarlet fever is a true childhood disease, usually seen between the ages of 2 to 10 years. It is caused by a Group A beta hemolytic streptococcal infection. The bacteria produces an erythrogenic toxin that is responsible for the rash. The child may get recurrent streptococcal infections but the rash only occurs once.

The disease is spread by direct exposure to an infected child. The child is contagious 24 hours before the symptoms of the streptococcal infection (usually a sore throat) and remains contagious up to three weeks. The incubation period is between three to five days.

HISTORY AND PHYSICAL EXAMINATION

Characteristically, the rash occurs three to four days after a history of a sore throat. Fever, nose bleeds, headache, and general malaise are frequently reported. On physical examination, there are often large, tender posterior cervical lymph nodes and exudate on the tonsils. Early in the illness, the tongue has a white coating and the papillae become red and swollen (strawberry tongue). Later in the illness, the white coating peels off and the tongue becomes more raspberry in color (raspberry tongue). Petechiae may be present on the hard palate.

The rash is a bright red maculopapular lesion with a fine sandpaper-like texture. This rash will blanch on pressure. Beginning at the base of the neck, the rash proceeds down the body in a linear pattern, and is less intense on the face, completely sparing the skin around the mouth. It is more prevalent under the axilla and in the genital area. The anticubital folds of the elbow may become dark red with fine petechiae. This is known as Pastia's sign and is diagnostic of scarlet fever. Toward the end of the illness, the rash begins to peel. The duration of the rash is between four to ten days.

DIAGNOSTIC TESTS

When presented with a classic case of scarlet fever, the value of performing a throat culture is debatable. However, in those cases where the signs and symptoms are less well-defined, a throat culture is warranted. To culture for Group A beta hemolytic *Streptococcus,* a blood agar media is used.

MANAGEMENT

Penicillin is the drug of choice for streptococcal infections. However, if an allergy to penicillin exists, erythromycin is the preferred medication.

STUDY QUESTIONS

Circle all that apply.

It is 9:30 AM on April 14th. John Dawney telephones your office regarding his 9-month-old daughter. He tells you that she has been sleeping more than usual and feels very hot. He is sure she has a fever but admits that he has not measured it with a thermometer. She is not interested in eating, but will take her milk and juices, if encouraged. He denies irritability, vomiting, or diarrhea.

1. You tell Mr. Dawney:

   a. to bring his daughter to the office
   b. to give his daughter aspirin to be repeated every four hours, and call back this afternoon is she is no better
   c. to measure his daughter's temperature and call you back
   d. to telephone his wife and tell her to come home because her daughter is ill

   It is now 3:30 PM and Mr. Dawney telephones your office (he did as requested in question 1). He is very concerned. His daughter's rectal temperature is 104.4° F and he gave her a second dose of aspirin two hours ago. He says that she sleeps continuously. When awake, she cries more than usual but continues to take her milk and juices well.
   The office is full of clients and you are 30 minutes behind schedule. Mr. Dawney is a competent parent.

2. You tell Mr. Dawney:

   a. to give his daughter acetaminophen now and then alternate it with aspirin every two hours; he is to call back if her temperature is not 100° F or less
   b. to telephone his wife and tell her to come home because her daughter is ill
   c. to give his daughter a tepid bath
   d. to bring his daughter to the office

It is the next day and Mr. Dawney telephones to say that his daughter's temperature was 105° F one hour ago. Presently it is 100.8° F. She had aspirin and a tepid bath about 45 minutes ago. During the night she developed a slight cough but no new symptoms. He is very worried and asks to see you.

3. You tell Mr. Dawney:

   a. to bring his daughter to your office
   b. that it is unnecessary to bring his daughter in if her temperature remains about 100° F
   c. to telephone his wife and tell her to come home because her daughter is ill
   d. to wait until tomorrow unless new symptoms occur; there are no appointments available today

You see Mr. Dawney's daughter in the office this afternoon. She is an alert, crying, 9-month-old girl who does not appear very ill. The physical examination is remarkable only for a rectal temperature of 102.2° F and enlarged occipital lymph nodes. This week there have been two other very young children in the office with similar clinical histories. On the third day of their illness, their temperatures dropped to normal and a rash appeared.

4. Based on this information, your best assessment is:

   a. an upper respiratory illness
   b. rubella
   c. roseola
   d. scarlet fever

5. Based on your assessment from question 4, you tell Mr. Dawney:

   a. to continue with the antipyretic and tepid baths but add an antihistamine
   b. to continue with the antipyretic and tepid baths but avoid pregnant women and large crowds
   c. to continue with the antipyretic and tepid baths and to expect the temperature to drop and his daughter to break out in a rash within the next 24 hours or so
   d. to continue with the antipyretic and tepid baths and to add penicillin

The next client is Ms. Jackson's 12-year-old son, Peter. He is in for a camp physical. During the history, you discover that Ms. Jackson's 6-year-old son has a mild case of chickenpox. According to Ms. Jackson,

Peter has never had chickenpox. This concerns Ms. Jackson and she asks if you would mind answering a few questions. You agree, and Ms. Jackson pulls a list from her handbag. The following are five of the questions she asked:

6. "My younger son's rash started yesterday. When can he return to school?"

   a. in about 10 days all the skin lesions will be gone and he can return to school
   b. when all the skin lesions are crusted over, he will no longer be contagious and he can return to school
   c. since this is a highly contagious disease, he should remain home for at least two weeks
   d. since the virus is spread from the respiratory tract, he can return to school once all his upper respiratory symptoms are gone

7. "Is there anything special I should be doing for my younger son?"

   a. keep his nails short and bathe him frequently
   b. if he has mouth lesions, give him a soft diet
   c. apply topical calamine lotion to help reduce itching
   d. apply topical steroid ointment to help reduce itching

8. "Since Peter has never had chickenpox, should I try to keep him away from his younger brother?"

   a. since chickenpox is not very contagious, Peter will probably not become ill
   b. the virus is shed from the respiratory tract and stool
   c. the virus is shed from the skin vesicles and urine
   d. since chickenpox is highly contagious, Peter will probably become ill

9. "Peter is going to camp in three weeks. Do you think we should try to postpone these arrangements?"

   a. no, the incubation period is 7 to 10 days and one is ill between 5 to 10 days
   b. no, the incubation period is 7 to 10 days and one is ill between 10 to 14 days
   c. yes, the incubation period is 10 to 21 days and one is ill between 5 to 10 days
   d. yes, the incubation period is 10 to 12 days and one is ill between 10 to 14 days

10. "If Peter does get chickenpox, what should I expect?"

    a. about 3 days before the rash, Peter may have a headache, fever (usually less than 102° F), sore throat, and poor appetite
    b. usually the rash will begin at the hairline
    c. since he is older, his symptoms may be more severe than your younger child's
    d. since he is older, his symptoms may be less severe than your younger child's

    Your next client is 4-year-old girl, Nancy Adams. Nancy is new to the office. Her mother tells you that Nancy has had a severe cold and a high fever (103° to 104° F) for the past two-and-a-half days. Ms. Adams says that she usually does not bring her daughter in for colds, but this time she looks sicker to her than she has ever seen.

11. Which of the following usually presents like Nancy's clinical history?

    a. measles
    b. roseola
    c. scarlet fever
    d. rubella

    You inquire about Nancy's immunizations. Ms. Adams shows you her daughter's immunization record.
    DPT, polio (2 months of age)
    DPT (4 months of age)
    DPT, polio (6 months of age)
    measles, mumps, rubella, (12 months of age)
    DPT, polio (24 months of age)

12. Is this an acceptable immunization record?

    a. yes
    b. yes, she will need a booster DPT and polio before she is 7 years old
    c. no, she missed a polio booster at age 4 months
    d. no, she needs the measles, mumps, rubella vaccination repeated

13. Nancy Adams' physical examination is remarkable for an oral temperature of 102.8° F, a mucopurulent nasal discharge, conjunctivitis, and red eruptions with white centers on the buccal mucosa. These are pathognomonic for measles. What are these eruptions called?

    a. Pastia's spots
    b. Koplik's spots
    c. rubeola spots
    d. strawberry spots

14. You advise Ms. Adams that the rash:

    a. will appear in less than 36 hours
    b. will appear in more than 36 hours
    c. will start at the hairline and neck
    d. will start on the trunk

15. Ms. Adams expects her sister's family for dinner early next week. Her sister has a 4-month-old daughter. You advise Ms. Adams to cancel the dinner and:

    a. explain that although the baby is probably passively protected, it is best not to expose the baby to measles
    b. inquire if Ms. Adams has ever had the measles
    c. explain that Nancy will be contagious until the fifth day of the rash
    d. explain that Nancy will be contagious for the next 10 days

    The final client of the day is Julia Harris. Julia is 17 years old and is in for a college entrance physical. During the history, she states that she has had measles and mumps but never rubella. According to her immunization record she has never received the rubella vaccine.

16. Your next step is:

    a. to obtain a rubella titer
    b. to give her the rubella vaccine
    c. to inquire if she is sexually active
    d. to advise her to get a rubella vaccine before she gets married

17. Julia Harris is very unhappy about receiving any vaccine. She protests loudly. You explain:

    a. that for those over 16 years old, rubella can produce very serious complications
    b. that if she becomes pregnant and gets rubella her baby can have severe malformations
    c. that rubella is highly contagious
    d. that if she gets rubella, she could give it to a pregnant woman

18. Which of the following is/are true about rubella?

    a. the incubation period is between 14 to 21 days
    b. the incubation period is between 7 to 14 days
    c. one is contagious 7 days before the rash until 7 days after the appearance of the rash
    d. one is contagious 3 to 4 days before the rash until the rash disappears

The receptionist tells you that Mr. Clark telephoned about his 3-year-old son. He is very concerned that the child might be having an allergic reaction to the penicillin you gave him three days ago. His son broke out in a rash today. After reviewing the son's chart, there is no history of scarlet fever or penicillin allergy.

19. Which of the following is/are true statement(s) regarding the rash of scarlet fever?

  a. the rash begins at the base of the neck and spreads downward
  b. the rash blanches and has a fine sandpaper-like texture
  c. the rash often spares the area around the mouth
  d. the rash is more prevalent on the trunk of the body

  Since you were unable to make an accurate assessment of the rash over the telephone, you plan to stop by Mr. Clark's house on your way home.

20. Which of the following physical findings would aid you in your assessment of scarlet fever?

  a. dark red lines with petechiae in the palmar folds of the elbow
  b. a white coating on the tongue with swollen red papillae
  c. petechiae on the hard palate
  d. a raspberry-colored tongue

21. As you suspected, Mr. Clark's son has scarlet fever. You advise Mr. Clark that:

  a. the rash will probably peel
  b. nosebleeds are not uncommon with scarlet fever
  c. his son will *never* have scarlet fever again
  d. for safety measures, you will switch his son from penicillin to erythromycin

ANSWERS

1. c	7. a, b, c
2. a, c	8. d
3. a	9. c
4. c	10. a, c
5. c	11. a, c
6. b	12. d

13. b

14. a, c

15. a, b, c

16. a, c

17. b, d

18. a, c

19. a, b, c

20. all of the above

21. a, b, c

BIBLIOGRAPHY

Hughes, J. G. *Synopsis of pediatrics,* (5th ed.). St. Louis: C. V. Mosby, 1980.

Kempe, C. H., et al. *Current pediatric diagnosis and treatment,* (7th ed.). Philadelphia: W. B. Saunders, 1980.

Krugman, S. and Ward, R. *Infectious Diseases of Children and Adults,* (7th ed.). St. Louis: C. V. Mosby, 1981.

Nelson, W. E. *Textbook of pediatrics.* Philadelphia: W. B. Saunders, 1975.

Report of the Committee on Infectious Diseases. *1977 The Red Book.* Evanston, Ill.: American Academy of Pediatrics.

CHAPTER 15

ORTHOPEDIC PROBLEMS

Martha Hudson Snow

The child who appears with an acute or insidious orthopedic problem is a frequent yet often perplexing challenge. The list of problems that appears ranges from minor trauma or common developmental deviations, which can be managed by the pediatric nurse practitioner, to complex and serious metabolic and infectious processes, which demand immediate referral. The most important aspect of pediatric orthopedics for the nurse practitioner, therefore, is the early detection of skeletal abnormalities and the investigation of orthopedic complaints to prevent further problems.

HISTORY

There is no substitute for a thorough health history when evaluating the child with a skeletal disturbance. The clinician should first obtain specific subjective information regarding the presenting symptom. This should include the type of pain; length of time that the symptom has been present; the exact site of pain if applicable; aggravating or alleviating factors, for example, positioning; and most important, a known history of trauma to the area of complaint.

One should also elicit information concerning birth and past medical history. Pertinent birth history would include presentation (especially breech), prematurity, congenital abnormalities, and birth injuries or insults (such as anoxia). A history of an antecedent or concurrent infectious process, especially of the respiratory tract or soft tissue, may prove to be vital information. Data regarding chronic illnesses, diet, present medicines, new footwear, and sleeping posture may provide significant guides to diagnosis. A family history of any skeletal abnormalities or metabolic disorders is also important.

Direct observation during the history taking and before commencing the physical examination may provide diagnostic clues. It is important to note the child's overall posturing and body alignment. The child may limp or a younger child may refuse to lie in a particular position. With the child seated, any muscle spasm or guarding should be noted.

PHYSICAL EXAMINATION

After the history is obtained, a complete physical examination should be performed, examining last that part that is symptomatic by history. Inspection of the musculoskeletal system progresses from the general to the specific, comparing sides for any asymmetries. The skin should be inspected for ecchymoses, puncture marks, scars, and discoloration. Signs of inflammation, such as erythema, swelling, warmth, and/or tenderness should be noted. Dimpling, a patch of hair, or hyper- or hypopigmented skin in the lumbosacral area may be a tip-off to a congenital spinal cord anomaly. Measurements may detect shortening or lengthening of an extremity and swelling or atrophy of a joint or muscle. Normal fat pads may be obliterated, signaling inflammation or soft tissue infection.

The bones are palpated noting the general shape and contour and also looking for warmth, tenderness, or pain with direct pressure. Pain may manifest itself by limited movement, the child's refusal to stand, or a limp when walking. While examining the bones and joints, the practitioner notes the child's facial expression and if crying is elicited. Active and passive range of motion should be the same for individual joints, with any limitation of motion carefully recorded. The strength of movement should be tested with symmetry of strength noted. At the conclusion of the examination, the cooperative child is requested to walk, run, squat, and stand on one leg.

DIAGNOSTIC TESTS

The diagnosis frequently can be made on the basis of history and physical findings; however, roentgenography may often be required to confirm a suspected diagnosis. In addition to the area of interest, an x-ray film of the opposite asymptomatic body part is generally taken for comparison. Certain ancillary laboratory data also may be needed for diagnosis, such as a complete blood count and sedimentation rate. The sedimentation rate (ESR) helps differentiate between systemic disease or infection and local trauma. The ESR increases in osteomyelitis, septic joint disease, rheumatoid arthritis, collagen disease, or malignancy. In trauma, the ESR remains normal.

CONGENITAL DEFORMITIES

Congenital Hip Dislocation

The incidence of congenital dislocation of the hip (CHD) is 10/1,000 live births in the United States. The etiology is both mechanical and physiologic. Tight maternal musculature, breech presentation, and hormonal influences all may play a role in the development of CHD. It is six times more frequent in females and appears to have a familial tendency.

Ortolani and Barlow maneuvers are the most clinically reliable methods for diagnosis of CHD. The Ortolani examination is a test of femur reduction. With the infant supine, the hips and knees are flexed while the examiner places the middle finger of one hand over the greater trochanter, and the thumb over the lesser trochanter. The pelvis is stabilized by the other hand. The thigh is lifted to mid-abduction while the thumb pressure is applied backward and outward over the lesser trochanter. The palpable "click" on entry or exit of the femoral head is clinically diagnostic.

The Barlow examination is the reverse of the Ortolani. With the infant's hips and knees flexed, the examiner applies pressure with the thumb in the region of the lesser trochanter. If the femoral head is unstable, this examination may dislocate it.

Other diagnostic findings of CHD are marked limitation of hip abduction, prominent trochanter, and flattened buttock on the affected side. Assymmetry of gluteal, popliteal, and inguinal skin folds may be noted, however, this is not always reliable. The goal of management is to reduce the hip, keeping the femoral head inside the acetabulum until reversal of the pathologic changes occurs. The earlier the reduction is accomplished, the better the prognosis. If the hip is reduced within the first year of life, it will appear normal on a roentgenogram and have normal function. Treatment of CHD after 12 months of age is not likely to result in a radiographically normal hip, and prognosis for normal hip function decreases with increasing age.

Metatarsus Adductus

Metatarsus adductus is a turning-in or adduction of the forefoot while the hindfoot remains in normal position. This foot deformity occurs quite commonly and is often associated with internal tibial torsion and an everted or flat foot. The origin is usually congenital due to abnormal uterine position.

Normally, a line drawn along the hindpart of the foot should extend through the second toe or between the second and third toe. In less severe cases (when the forefoot can be abducted past the midline, but less than 30°) stretching exercises are performed at diaper change by holding the heel in a neutral position while moving the forefoot into abduction, where it is held for a count of five, then repeated five times. It is advisable not to allow the infant to sleep face down with the feet curled in. While some authorities suggest reversing shoes, this is controversial since the toes may be pushed over and initiate a new foot problem. If the deformity is not corrected by stretching exercises within three to four months, referral is appropriate. The prognosis is not good if the forepart of the foot cannot be moved beyond the neutral point. These infants should be referred and treatment started within the first few weeks of life.

Club Foot

Club foot is a common foot deformity with an incidence of 2/1,000 live births. It occurs two times more frequently in boys than in girls. The most common form of club foot is the equinovarus deformity which represents approximately 95% of cases. This disfigurement has three features: inversion of the heel, adduction of the forepart of the foot, and planter flexion of the foot.

On examination, it is important to distinguish between positional equinovarus due to intrauterine posture, which can be readily placed in a normal position, and true clubfoot, which cannot be placed in a neutral position. Early recognition is critical and treatment is usually initiated shortly after birth when the joints are maximally flexible. Treatment consisting of manipulation and casting or surgery is usually quite successful. This foot deformity recurs in approximately half of children, therefore, follow-up is important until their growth is complete.

ACQUIRED DISORDERS

Legg-Calvé-Perthes Disease

Legg-Calvé-Perthes disease is an avascular necrosis (deterioration and regeneration of one or more ossification centers without infection) of the femoral area. It usually occurs in children ages 4 to 8 years. There seems to be some correlation between this disease and a low birth weight. The first symptom is a limp, usually accompanied by pain in the hip or referral to the knee. The one-sided limp is characterized by quick, soft steps to shorten the period of weight-bearing on the involved leg. Symptoms may have been present for months before professional advice is sought. On examination, the range of motion of the hip is limited, with tenderness over the anterior capsule. Measurement of the thighs and calves may reveal atrophy on the affected side. Referral is warranted if there is any suspicion of this disorder. The progress is good in children less than 5 years of age, fair in ages 5 to 7 years, and poor in children over 7. The goal of treatment is to prevent deformity of the femoral head and prevent degenerative changes in the hip. Management may range from confinement to bed to bracing, casting, or surgery.

Osgood-Schlatter's Disease

Osgood-Schlatter's disease involves pain and swelling of the tibial tubercle at the insertion of the patellar tendon. This disorder occurs most frequently in boys between the ages of 10 and 15 years. The child may complain of knee pain that is aggravated by excessive activity. On examination, the knee is swollen and tender to direct pressure. Pain may be reproduced by extending the knee against resistance. These children should be referred to an orthopedist. The goal of treatment is to decrease stress at the tubercle, usually accomplished by four to six weeks restriction from strenuous physical activity or by casting to rest the knee.

Painful Hip

The differential diagnosis for the child who appears with hip pain varies from minor trauma to life-threatening illnesses. The most important causes to recognize and rule out are the bone and joint infections—osteomyelitis and septic arthritis. Legg-Calvé-Perthes disease, discussed earlier, often is accompanied by hip pain. Although not a devastating disease, the most common cause of painful hip in children is probably acute transient synovitis.

Osteomyelitis. Osteomyelitis is an infection commonly originating as a hematogenous abscess in the metaphysis of long bones. It most often occurs in children of less than 10 years and is found twice as frequently in boys. The predominant organism is *Staphylococcus aureus*. Children with osteomyelitis are usually systemically ill with high fever and other signs of sepsis. The affected bone sites are usually extremely painful.

Several distinguishing features may help differentiate osteomyelitis from other acute infections. Swelling is a prominent and almost constant feature of osteomyelitis with maximum swelling around the affected area. Tenderness is maximum over the metaphysis. If handled carefully, joint motion is surprisingly good with little pain.

The importance of early recognition and referral of osteomyelitis cannot be overemphasized. Laboratory findings may or may not be helpful. The sedimentation rate frequently is elevated while leukocytosis may or may not be present. Blood cultures and an aspirate of soft tissue, bone, or both should be obtained before instituting antibiotic therapy. Roentgenographic findings may not be apparent for 10 to 15 days after the appearance of symptoms. Bone scintigrams after injection of a radioactive nucleotide can differentiate among cellulitis, osteomyelitis, and pyarthrosis.

If osteomyelitis is clinically suspected, the child should be referred for definitive diagnosis immediately. Hospitalization and 6 to 12 weeks of appropriate antibiotics is usually indicated.

Septic Arthritis (Pyarthrosis).   Septic arthritis is a bacterial joint disease seen most commonly in toddlers of 1 to 2 years of age who have recently had an upper respiratory or skin infection. The hip is involved most often in infants and is second in frequency to the knee in toddlers. *S. aureus* is the frequent causative agent in older children whereas *Hemophilus influenzae* is common under 2 to 3 years of age. The infected joint is warm and swollen with maximal tenderness over the joint line. Here, unlike osteomyelitis, pain is exacerbated by passive motion or increased pressure in the affected joint. Another distinguishing characteristic is the limitation of joint motion. Classically, there is an elevated white count and sedimentation rate.

Diagnosis is best made by arthrocentesis. Septic arthritis, especially in the hip joint, is a surgical emergency. If more than three or four days pass before treatment is begun, it is too late to prevent irreparable damage. Therefore, prompt referral is crucial.

Acute Transient Synovitis.   Acute transient synovitis is a self-limiting unilateral condition of the hip joint lasting from a few days to two to three weeks. It is probably the most common orthopedic condition causing a limp in the otherwise normal child. The exact cause of this condition is unknown, but minor trauma has been known to be implicated. It affects mainly children less than 10 years of age, and occurs more frequently in boys.

Diagnosis of transient synovitis is one of exclusion. The differential diagnosis is primarily with septic arthritis. Unlike septic arthritis, the child with transient synovitis is not ill, there is an absence of systemic symptoms, and relatively good range of motion of the joint. Laboratory findings are usually benign. The goal of treatment is the relief of pain. Management consists of bed rest for seven to ten days, local application of heat and massage of the hip area, and aspirin.

Juvenile Rheumatoid Arthritis

Juvenile rheumatoid arthritis (JRA) is a disease characterized by chronic synovitis and extraarticular manifestations. The onset varies considerably from involvement of one joint without systemic symptoms and multiple joint involvement with or without systemic manifestations, to an acute febrile onset with polyarthritis. Persistent arthritis of a single joint for two or three consecutive months is considered to be diagnostic of juvenile rheumatoid arthritis. Significant differentiating findings in this disease are its slower onset, greater range of motion in joints, and tenderness primarily over the joint and not the metaphysis. Juvenile rheumatoid arthritis often is confused with septic arthritis or rheumatic fever but it rarely appears as acutely as these conditions. The laboratory findings are usually within normal limits or nonspecific. Positive agglutination tests for rheumatoid factors are rarely found in children before the age of 8 years.

Scoliosis

Scoliosis is a lateral deviation of the spinal column from the midline that may or may not include rotation or deformity of the vertebrae. It may be classified as a structural or nonstructural type. Nonstructural scoliosis may be due to positive or compensatory causes, such as a discrepancy in leg lengths. Structural scoliosis may be idiopathic, congenital, or due to neuromuscular causes, such as polio, cerebral palsy, or muscular dystrophy. Seventy percent of all cases of scoliosis are idiopathic. Idiopathic scoliosis occurs seven times more frequently in girls, most commonly from 10 years of age to the age of bone maturity. There also seems to be a familial tendency.

Children between the ages of 8 and 15 should be routinely screened for scoliosis. The child is examined preferably in underwear. The child's trunk alignment is observed from the front, side, and back while standing erect and as the child bends forward, symmetry of shoulders, scapulae, posterior rib cage, flanks, and hips is noted. With the child standing erect, a plumb line or tape measure is dropped from the occiput. Normally, the head is centered exactly over the gluteal cleft. Any deformity noted requires referral to an orthopedist to prevent any progression of the problem. Management may include a Milwaukee brace, traction, casting, or surgery.

Slipped Capital Femoral Epiphysis

Slipped capital femoral epiphysis (adolescent coxa vara) is a mechanical displacement of the epiphyseal plate occurring most often in the overweight adolescent boy. Forty percent of cases involve both hips. The etiology is unknown and the onset is usually insidious. The child often limps, with the foot on the involved side externally rotated. The hip motion is limited and hip pain may be referred to the knee. The diagnosis can be confirmed on roentgenogram. The earlier the diagnosis, the better the prognosis. The goal of therapy is to arrest the slipping of the epiphysis by immobilizing the hip.

The most reliable therapy is surgery but a short plaster boot to both legs with a cross bar or a hip spica cast has been used.

Battered Child Syndrome

It should be mentioned that it is not uncommon for the battered child to have musculoskeletal symptoms. When trauma is suspected but cannot be explained in a young child, and other symptoms, such as bruising, are present, child abuse should be suspected. Roentgenograms of the long bones and chest can lead to recognition of this syndrome. The diagnostic hallmark of the battered child is multiple occult metaphyseal fractures in various stages of repair. Suspected cases of child abuse should be reported to the appropriate agency.

DEVELOPMENTAL DEVIATIONS

Bowlegs and Knock Knees

Bowlegs, or genu varum, occurs as a normal physiologic variation from 12 to 18 months of age. The evaluation should include a family history and leg measurements for inequality and asymmetry. The distance between the medial aspects of knees when the medial malleoli are held against each other, should also be measured. Normally, this distance is approximately 1½ inches, and bowing that is greater than this should be referred for treatment, usually with a Denis-Browne splint. Physiologic genu varum, on the other hand, generally straightens spontaneously with growth. The child is usually followed at regular well child visits and the parents are reassured.

Knock knees, also called genu valgum, is commonly caused by hypermobility of the knee joint. It occurs as a normal physiologic phenomenon in children ages 2 to 7 years and is generally ignored in this age group unless it is excessive, asymmetrical, or accompanied by shortened stature. The distance between the malleoli with the medial aspects of the knees held against each other should be measured. If this distance is 3 inches or less in the 2 to 5 year-old child, the valgum will improve spontaneously. The aim of treatment, if needed, is to prevent further stretching of the collateral ligaments. Children should avoid the "TV position" (squatting with the buttocks on the floor and the knees and ankles flexed flat against the floor), which further stretches those ligaments.

Genu varum or valgum that is extreme but symmetrical may be due to a metabolic or endocrine disease, whereas unilateral or asymmetrical varum or valgum may be associated with tumors, congenital deformities, or trauma. Other causes of varum or valgum include Blount's disease (or growth disturbance of the tibia), rickets, and trauma.

Pes Planus

Pes planus, more commonly called flat feet, occurs when the arch of the foot appears flat on the floor with weight bearing. In children from 2 to 3 years of age, flexible flat feet are caused by hypermobility of the joints. In these cases, the flat arch disappears when toe walking. A plantar fat pad is normal until 2 or 3 years of age. No treatment is required other than reassurance to parents. Rigid flat feet may be due to a tightness of the heel cord. Although rigid flat feet are uncommon, one should look for dorsal and plantar flexion of the heel to rule out this deformity.

Internal Tibial Torsion

A common condition causing intoeing is internal tibial torsion. Often, this medial twisting of the tibia is not noted until the child begins to walk. On examination, the feet turn inward in both the supine and standing position with normal hip rotation. This deformity may be associated with metatarsus varus or genu varum. Correction is usually required if the leg is externally rotated 30 to 35°. It is best to initiate treatment by 18 months of age. Treatment by the orthopedist depends on the age of the child and the severity of the deformity, and may range from passive stretching exercises or night splints to corrective casting or surgery. In mild or early cases, a change in sleeping position from supine to prone or to the side may be recommended.

Medial Femoral Torsion

Medial femoral torsion (increased femoral anteversion) is frequently a cause of intoeing seen in children ages 3 to 7 years. This condition is usually bilaterally symmetrical and is more commonly seen in girls. The prominent feature on physical examination is the limited lateral rotation of the hips in the extended position. Generally, the condition disappears spontaneously, rarely requiring treatment.

Management

Management of most of the above problems for the pediatric nurse practitioner is early recognition and referral to an orthopedist for manipulation, casting, bracing, or surgery. The nurse practitioner may often be involved in the follow-up care, which includes parent counseling, use of special shoes, and cast care.

Counseling. Counseling is very important in the management of musculoskeletal problems in children. Since the nurse practitioner may be the first to suspect an orthopedic problem, he or she will often need to provide the initial counseling. Of course parents need to receive information concerning the child's specific problem and understand the importance of the referral. Many parents may have feelings of guilt or inadequacy, especially if the child has a birth deformity. Clarification of the problem and allowing the parents to discuss their feelings and concerns may help reduce anxiety and guilt. Being available on an ongoing basis to provide reassurance or to answer parents' questions helps the family to cope more effectively with the orthopedic problem.

Shoes.   In general, the normal shoe in childhood should be of ample size, well-ventilated, flexible, and inexpensive. Tennis shoes, booties, or fabric shoes are recommended for the normal foot in infancy because they allow full motion of the feet. Some toddlers may require high-topped shoes to keep the shoe on the foot. Corrective shoes and shoe modifications may be recommended by the pediatric orthopedist for metatarsus adductus or intoeing due to medial tibial torsion, for leg length inequalities, or to manage extreme bowlegs, knock knees, or flat feet.

Cast Care.   When a child is immobilized in a cast, the parents may need support and advice regarding cast care. The aim of casting is to protect, immobilize, and support a part of the musculoskeletal system or to reposition or maintain alignment. Parents should be instructed in appropriate cast and skin care. They should notify the clinic if the child develops a fever, a musty unpleasant odor from the cast, a relative coldness of the dependent part, or pain—increasing, persistent, and localized. Whenever possible, the normalcy of the child should be stressed in familial and social interactions in spite of the cast.

STUDY QUESTIONS

Circle all that apply.

A 6 year-old boy appears with a limp, noted initially by his mother about two weeks ago. She became concerned yesterday when the child began to cry and complain of pain.

1. Of the following, which would be included in your initial differential diagnosis?

   a. acute transient synovitis
   b. Legg-Calvé-Perthes disease
   c. septic arthritis
   d. osteomyelitis

2. Physical exam is significant only for limited ROM of the hip. No systemic illness noted. No fever. Lab data is unavailable. Your plan would include:

    a. obtain x-ray films
    b. refer to appropriate resource
    c. hospitalize immediately
    d. initiate appropriate antibiotics

3. Match the lab data with the diagnosis.

    (1) acute transient synovitis
    (2) Legg Calvé-Perthes disease
    (3) osteomyelitis
        a. $\pm \uparrow$ sed rate, $\pm \uparrow$ WBC
        b. $\uparrow$ sed rate, $\uparrow$ WBC
        c. sed rate normal, WBC normal

4. The predominant organism in osteomyelitis is:

    a. *Hemophilus influenza*
    b. *Staphylococcus aureus*
    c. Group A *Streptococcus*
    d. *Staphylococcus epidermidis*

5. *Routine* screening for scoliosis includes:

    a. assessing symmetry of shoulders, scapulae, posterior rib cage, flanks, hips
    b. roentgenograms or dorsal spine
    c. noting trunk alignment while standing erect and bending forward
    d. dropping a plumb line from occiput noting if centered over the gluteal cleft

6. When counseling the parent of a child with the clubbing of the feet, the nurse practitioner should include:

    a. appropriate cast care
    b. stress the normality of the child although he or she will require special surgery and care shortly after birth
    c. try to alleviate parental feelings of guilt and inadequacy due to birth anomaly
    d. stress importance of follow-up with recurrence

7. *Immediate* orthopedic referrals include:

    a. a 3-year-old with minimal knock knees
    b. a 3-year-old with unilateral bowleg
    c. a 2-year-old with flexible flat feet
    d. a 3-month-old with internal tibial torsion

8. An important factor in the development of congenital hip dislocation is:

   a. tight maternal musculature
   b. breech presentation
   c. hormonal influences
   d. all of above

ANSWERS

1. a, b, d   4. b
2. a, b   5. a, c, d
3. (1) a   6. a, b, c, d
   (2) c   7. b
   (3) b   8. d

BIBLIOGRAPHY

Ahronheim, G. A. Common bacterial infections in infancy and childhood infections of the skeletal system. *Drugs, 16,* 1978, 210–218.

Cohen, J. Skeletal problems of children. *Hospital Practice,* 1977, *12, 7,* 77–89.

Chung, S. Diseases of the developing hip joint. *Pediatric Clinics of North America,* 1977, *24, 4,* 857–870.

Hensinger, R. N. Congenital dislocation of the hip. *Clinical Symposia,* 1979, *31,* 1.

Holt de Toledo, C. The patient with scoliosis: the defect, classification and detection. *American Journal of Nursing,* 1979, *79, 9,* 1588–1591.

Kaye, J. J. Roentgenographic evaluation of children with acute onset of a limp. *Pediatric Annals,* 1976, *1,* 11–30.

Keim, H. A. Scoliosis. *Clinical Symposia,* 1978, *30,* 1.

Kempe, C. H., Silverman, F. N., & Steele, B. F. The battered-child syndrome. *Journal of the American Medical Association,* 1962, *181, 1,* 17–24.

Larson, C. B., & Gould, M. Orthopedic nursing. St. Louis: C. V. Mosby, 1978.

McDade, W. Bowlegs & knock knees. *Pediatric Clinics of North America,* 1977, *24, 4,* 825–839.

Mitchell, G. P. Orthopaedic problems in children. *The Practitioner,* 1979, *222,* 46–54.

Salter, R. B. Common normal variations in the musculoskeletal system. *Textbook of disorders and injuries of the musculoskeletal system.* Baltimore: Williams and Wilkins, 1970.

Salter, R. B. Congenital abnormalities. *Textbook of disorders and injuries of the musculoskeletal system.* Baltimore: Williams and Wilkins, 1970.

Schaller, J. G. Arthritis and infection of bones and joints. *Pediatric Clinics of North America,* 1977, *24, 4,* 775–790.

Singer, J. Evaluation of acute and insidious gait disturbance in children less than five years of age. *Advances in Pediatrics,* 1979, *26,* 209–273.

Staheli, L. T., & Griffin, L. Corrective shoes for children: a survey of current practice. *Pediatrics,* 1980, *65, 1,* 13–17.

Staheli, L. T. Torsional deformity. *Pediatric Clinics of North America,* 1977, *24, 4,* 799–811.

Vaughan, V. C., McKay, R. J. Jr., & Behrman, R. E. *Nelson's textbook of pediatrics.* Philadelphia: W. B. Saunders, 1979.

VuQuoc, D., Nelson, J. D., & Haltalin, K. C. Osteomyelitis in infants and children. *American Journal of Diseases of Children,* 1975, *129,* 1273–1278.

CHAPTER **16**

ADOLESCENCE

John W. Greene

Adolescence is a time of transition from childhood to adulthood. The adolescent is rapidly changing both physically and emotionally. Traditionally, adolescence has been defined as the period of life beginning at puberty and ending with the completion of growth. In recent years this has been broadened and now ranges from age 10 to 12 years to the early 20s.

The adolescent growth spurt is dramatic evidence of physical development. It begins in girls between 10.5 and 12 years of age and in boys between 12.5 and 15 years of age. During the years of peak height velocity, growth may be up to 12 cm per year. Normally, yearly weight gain parallels that of height. This growth spurt is accomplished by the actions of growth hormones and adrogens. It is important to note that adolescents vary widely from one another in the timing of their growth. The progression, however, is generally similar in all.

The body changes at puberty result from the release of gonadotrophin-releasing hormones secreted by the hypothalamus. These hormones stimulate the pituitary gland to produce gonadotrophins (LH and FSH). Luteinizing hormone and follicle-stimulating hormone in turn stimulate the gonads (ovaries in girls and testes in boys). The sex hormones produced by the gonads are responsible for secondary sexual maturation.

Tanner has charted the progression and sequence of these physical changes. The sequence is similar in all young people of the same sex, but the age at which they occur varies among individuals (1). In girls, the first evidence of puberty is breast development (thelarche). Breast budding generally begins as height velocity begins to increase. Breast development is followed closely by growth of pubic and axillary hair (adrenarche). Menarche (onset of menses) is generally last in the sequence. Onset of menses usually occurs after peak height velocity has been reached and stage three to four breast development has been attained (See Table 16.1).

Table 16.1. Usual Progression of Physical Development in Girls

Increased height
Breast budding (thearche)
Growth of public and axillary hair (adrenarche)
Peak height velocity (most rapid growth)
Onset of menses (menarche)

In boys, as shown in Table 16.2, testicular enlargement (from gonadotrophin stimulation) is usually the first evidence of secondary sexual development. This enlargement is associated with increased height. This is followed closely by increased pubic, axillary and facial hair, and penile enlargement. Height and weight changes in boys appear at a later chronologic age than in girls, but ultimately boys are taller and heavier. Body fat distribution parallels other secondary sexual changes in both sexes.

In addition to the physical changes that are occurring, adolescents are also experiencing dramatic emotional, intellectual, and social development. This development is marked by a striving to separate from family. Separation is necessary for adolescents to establish independence and identity. In addition, as illustrated in Table 16.3, the development of relationships and value systems, and acceptance of sexuality are major goals of adolescent psychosocial development. In attaining these goals, some turbulence may be encountered by each adolescent, and some will experience much more turmoil than others. As with physical development, girls mature psychosocially one to two years earlier than boys.

It may be useful to divide emotional development into stages and characterize each. In early adolescence (10 to 13 years), teenagers first discover that they are separate entities from their parents. This individualization process may be perceived by parent and teenager as a loss of established bonds between the two. When perceived in this manner, there may be alternating periods of closeness and rebellious behavior. This behavior may be difficult for parents to understand and emotionally unsettling for the teenager.

During middle adolescence (13 to 16 years), the separation process continues, and self-concept and identity formation begins. The peer group becomes very important during this stage, and fears of peer rejection produce a

Table 16.2. Usual Progression of Physical Development in Boys

Increased height
Testicular enlargement
Growth of pubic and axillary hair
Enlargement of the penis
Peak height velocity (most rapid growth)

Table 16.3. Developmental Tasks of Adolescence

Overall task
Establish identity
Other tasks
Establish independence
Establish comfort with body and sexuality
Build new relationships
Develop a workable value system
Develop career or vocational goals

need to look and act similar to peers. Same sex attachments, which are common in early adolescence, gradually give way to heterosexual alliances during middle adolescence.

In late adolescence (16 to 19 years), relationships established during middle adolescence form a basis for long-term commitments and caring relationships. Late adolescents also begin to resolve conflicting feelings about parents, and individualization with identity crystallization occurs. New considerations are given to career decisions and life goals as the adolescent approaches young adulthood.

A working knowledge of this developmental process is essential for professionals working with adolescents and their families. Anticipatory guidance regarding common problems encountered during the adolescent years should be started by age 11 to 12. Discussions with parents and teenagers should include nutrition, sexuality, drug use and abuse, accident prevention, school, expressions of emotions, peer relationships, and career plans.

HISTORY TAKING

Obtaining a complete history when interviewing teenage clients usually requires time with the adolescent alone, as well as time with parent and teenager together. Initially, it is desirable to see them together. This allows parents to give pertinent information, and to voice any concerns they might have. In addition, interaction between family members can be observed. After this initial interview, the adolescent should be interviewed alone. This is essential to obtain complete information, especially in the areas of sexuality and possible alcohol or drug use. When teenagers are approached in an objective manner, information can generally be obtained in potentially sensitive areas.

The adolescent's social history should also include information about peer relationships, school, extracurricular activities, dating, part-time jobs, and career plans. This information will aid in determining how well the teenager is advancing toward achieving the goals of adolescent development and taking responsibility for self.

PHYSICAL EXAMINATION

Adolescents should be given the option of having a parent in the room during the exam. Most adolescents over age 12 will choose to have parents wait outside. Many will have some degree of anxiety about even a routine exam, especially when the examiner is of the opposite sex. This anxiety can be reduced to a minimum by approaching the client in a calm and objective manner. In relieving anxiety, it is helpful to carry on a conversation with the adolescent while proceeding with the exam. The client's modesty must always be respected, but when indicated, a complete examination, including genital exam, must be performed.

The general examination is little different from that for an adult. One difference, however, is that growth and sexual development should be assessed routinely. This staging may be important in determining the timing of developmental events. In female adolescents, a pelvic examination should be performed when the client is sexually active, or when there are signs are symptoms of gynecologic problems. Routine pelvic examination in the nonsexually active and otherwise healthy adolescent female is not indicated until age 19 to 20.

DIAGNOSTIC TESTS

Few laboratory tests are routinely indicated in adolescents. It is clear that a routine hematocrit determination should be performed after onset of menses in adolescent girls, but its utility in boys is unproven. Although commonly performed, routine urinalysis in teenagers is of no proven value. This is also true for routine screening urine cultures. Screening cultures for gonorrhea are indicated for sexually active girls, and recent evidence suggests screening may be warranted in boys. Screening for blood lipid abnormalities is indicated in adolescents with close relatives who have atherosclerotic cardiovascular disease at an early age. Screening for scoliosis is a part of the routine physical exam in this age group. Immunizations should be updated with a tetanus-diphtheria (Td) booster given at age 14 to 15 years and every 10 years thereafter. Tuberculin skin testing is indicated biannually in low-risk populations and yearly in higher risk persons.

ADOLESCENT SEXUALITY AND CONTRACEPTION

Adolescents are generally candid about sexual activity when interviewed alone and approached objectively. Opportune times to discuss this subject are while taking a social history (peers, boy-girlfriend, dating), and when performing routine genitourinary examinations.

It is currently estimated 50% of both boys and girls are sexually active by age 19. This represents a clear increase in teenage sexual activity (based on comparison data from 10 years earlier). The increase in sexual activity, poor contraceptive practices, and declining marriage rates for teenagers have resulted in increased premarital pregnancies and out-of-wedlock births. While contraceptive use has increased, use of effective contraceptives are often delayed for over a year after beginning sexual activity. Major reasons cited for not using effective contraceptive methods include misinformation unexpected intercourse, and a lack of motivation to prevent pregnancy.

CONTRACEPTION FOR TEENAGERS

Oral Contraceptives

The high potential effectiveness of oral contraceptives (OCs) makes them the most commonly used method by teenagers, and current information indicates that this effectiveness is accompanied by only a minor risk of severe pill-related complications. As with persons of any age in whom OCs are being considered, a careful history and complete physical examination must be performed. This includes a pelvic examination, pap test, and a screening cervical culture for gonorrhea.

Clinicians should be familiar with all contraindications and potential side effects before prescribing OCs. In addition to the contraindications that apply to all women, OCs are contraindicated in teenagers who have not yet established regular menstrual cycles, and in those who have not yet completed their somatic growth.

When a decision is made to begin OCs, a combination pill containing 50 μg or less of estrogen is preferable. Numerous "low dosage" combination pills are available and effective. A major side effect of very low dosage pills is breakthrough bleeding and irregular menses. Teenagers should be informed of these possibilities and reassured that cycles will generally regulate within two to three months. This information may enhance compliance and continuation of use. Compliance may also be improved by prescribing a 28-day pill and scheduling frequent follow-up visits. We recommend return visits at one, three, and six months after beginning OCs. Follow-up evaluations of blood pressure, weight, and other potential side effects are similar to those in all women.

Condoms

Condoms are not a popular method of contraception among teenage boys in this country, but they have at least three major advantages as a method of choice for teens: (*a*) there are essentially no side effects; (*b*) they provide protection from common venereal diseases; and (*c*) they can be purchased without a prescription. Condoms are also the cheapest form of contraception for teenagers whose sex lives are sporadic. Educational efforts for teenagers should stress these facts, and teens choosing this method should be instructed in proper use.

Diaphragms

While the diaphragm is an effective method of birth control when used properly, few younger teenagers use it effectively. Many are uncomfortable with insertion and others feel that insertion interferes with the spontaneity of their relationship. Older and more motivated teenagers may choose this method and use it effectively.

Intrauterine Devices (IUD)

The IUD is an effective contraceptive method for adolescents, but recent reports indicate that pelvic inflammatory disease is five-to-ten times more common in adolescents using IUDs (when compared to older women using the same method). The risk of infection and subsequent risk of infertility must also be considered when prescribing IUDs for teenagers. When used, small devices, such as the copper seven, are usually selected.

Abstinence or "Saying No"

Self-assertion and the right to say no to sexual activity should always be discussed as an option for teenagers. This point can be made on an individual basis in the office or when assisting with sex education courses in schools.

ADOLESCENT PREGNANCY AND CHILDBIRTH

An estimated one million pregnancies occur in adolescents annually in the United States (2). Of these, 80% are reported to be unintended. The younger the teenager, the more likely that her pregnancy was unintended, and the higher the risk of complications for mother and infant when the pregnancy is carried to term. While many adolescent pregnancies are terminated by abortions, a large number of teenagers do not come to health care facilities until the second or even third trimester of pregnancy. This often makes them ineligible for simple and safe abortions. Late presentation also places them and their infants at higher risk for complications when they choose to carry the baby.

Pregnant teenagers should be strongly encouraged to seek prenatal care early, since recent data indicate that comprehensive prenatal care can significantly reduce complications of pregnancy and delivery. Others have also reported reduced numbers of repeat pregnancies in teenagers when contraceptive services are made available at the same site as prenatal services.

The number and rate of births declined during the 1970s for all teenagers except those less than 15 years of age. This group is at highest risk for complications, and also least likely to be able to care for a child. Once these teenage mothers give birth, almost all now keep their children in the household with them. There are an estimated 1.3 million children living with 1.1 million adolescent mothers in this country. A majority of these adolescent mothers live with their own parents or grandparents and receive much-needed financial and emotional support in this way.

Developmentally, children of adolescents appear to fare as well as those of older women when family support is available to them.

BEHAVIOR PROBLEMS

A frequent parental complaint is that the teenager is "difficult" or "won't mind." When presented with this complaint, the task of the health care provider is to determine whether the behavior is part of a normal adolescent need to establish independence or whether it represents true "out of control behavior" (3). In these situations, parents may need to be reminded that it is typical for teenagers to express opinions, argue their points, and protest what they consider unfair treatment. Although parents may feel stressed and out of control during these situations, reassurance and support is often all that is needed.

A key factor in aiding parents with "difficult" teenagers is helping them reestablish communication with their adolescent. This requires that parents set aside time for the teenager for sharing views. Parents also should be encouraged to set clear limits for behavior and define the consequences of transgressions. Although teens must be expected to test these limits, the stated consequences must follow when rules are broken. Idle parental threats are destructive to the parent-teenager relationship.

Normal independence-seeking behavior must be differentiated from behavior that may indicate severe adjustment difficulties. For example, delinquency, school failure, sexual promiscuity, alcohol and drug abuse, and self-destructive acts indicate major adjustment problems. When these behaviors are seen, intervention by a mental health professional will probably be needed. If a referral is made in the primary care provider should maintain involvement with the teenager and family.

ALCOHOL AND DRUG ABUSE

Alcohol and marijuana are commonly referred to as social drugs. They are also the drugs most commonly used and abused by teenagers. Although both are becoming socially acceptable in our society only alcohol is legal.

Alcohol use is common among teenagers, with an estimated 50% of high school students drinking at least occasionally and an estimated 30% classified as heavy drinkers. True problem drinkers account for only 15 to 20% of high school students, but this percentage is thought to be increasing. A "problem drinker" is defined as one who reports being drunk four or more times in the past year and/or encountered two or more negative consequences of drinking (trouble with teachers, peers, parents, or law enforcement agencies).

HISTORY

Teenagers who are experiencing difficulties with alcohol and/or marijuana rarely seek help of their own volition. They are either coerced into seeking help by parents or referred to health care professionals by schools or juvenile authorities. Drug use often begins as early as age 11 and usually as experimentation. Early use may give way to recreational use, and in a small percentage of youths, habitual use and abuse follows. Teenagers may be suspected of using drugs by parents or school officials because of disruptive behavior, changing moods, poor grades, truancy, or attending school while intoxicated. After being referred or coerced into seeking help, the adolescent often resents and resists the professional's attempts to intervene. This can usually be minimized by assuring the client that the provider will not act as a judge or parent figure.

PHYSICAL EXAMINATION

The examination is generally normal unless the client is acutely intoxicated. Acute alcohol intoxication is usually associated with poor coordination, slurred speech, and an alcoholic breath. The conjunctiva may be injected and the face flushed. The physical signs of marijuana intoxication include reddened conjunctiva, accelerated heart rate, and mildly elevated blood pressure. With both drugs, mood is altered. Marijuana also commonly produces a "light mood" or high, an altered perception of the environment, and laughter without provocation. The stigmata of chronic alcohol abuse are rare in adolescents and the effects of chronic marijuana use are largely unknown. Chronic respiratory complaints are common in heavy marijuana users.

MANAGEMENT

In experimental users, objective information should be provided to parents and teenagers on the consequences of heavy use. Scare tactics do not seem to be helpful, but facts, such as the effects of marijuana on the lung (worse than tobacco), decreased motor performance while under the influence of either drug, and the legality of use can be stressed. Decreased motor performance is especially significant since the most common cause of death in adolescents is accidental (automobile accidents). Recreational or habitual users may need referral to professionals specializing in drug treatment and rehabilitation.

OBESITY

Obesity is a common problem during adolescence, and studies indicate that obese adolescents are likely to carry this condition into their adult lives.

Most obese adolescents also suffer difficulties with poor self-esteem and body image at some time. It is common to have an obese adolescent, especially a girl, ask for an excuse from gym class to avoid the embarrassing experience of "dressing out" for gym.

HISTORY AND PHYSICAL EXAMINATION

A complete history and physical examination should be performed with particular attention to previous heights and weights. A careful dietary history will usually reveal excessive caloric intake, since most adolescent obesity is exogenous (overeating). Although organic causes are uncommon, they must be considered and ruled out by appropriate testing. A useful indicator in screening for an organic versus exogenous etiology is a comparison of height and weight. Obese adolescents whose height exceeds the 50% range rarely have organic (endocrine) causes for their obesity. Short stature and associated obesity, in contrast, suggest an organic etiology.

Several criteria for defining obesity have been proposed, but in most cases the diagnosis will be obvious to both clinician and client. It may be useful, however, to list the criteria commonly used. These include: a body weight either more than 10% in excess of the calculated normal or $\geq$ 90th percentile for persons of a given age, height, and sex. Skin fold measurements of adipose tissue are probably the most scientific way to quantitate obesity, but are not regularly used in clinical settings.

MANAGEMENT

After a diagnosis of exogenous obesity has been established, the basic approaches to management include: (*a*) caloric restriction (decreased caloric input); (*b*) physical exercise (increased caloric expenditure); and (*c*) behavior modification. Caloric restriction with a regular exercise program is needed for adolescents who have developed poor eating habits and sedentary lifestyles. Other teenagers who overeat because of stressful situations may require individual or family counseling. In either case, support from the teenager's family and/or another group is a useful adjunct to the weight-reduction program.

Behavior modification has also been used successfully in overweight teenagers. It involves making clients aware of their eating habits and the circumstances antecedent to their eating. After this is done, controlled eating is emphasized and mastered. Finally, the focus is changed to weight loss. Setting goals for weight loss, with periodic weight checks to evaluate progress, is helpful. Weekly checks are generally needed for the first two months. It should be emphasized that for any program to be successful, adolescent clients must have a desire to lose weight. Maintainence of weight loss generally requires some modification in life-style.

ACNE

Acne is one of the most common and troublesome physical problems encountered during adolescence. It affects nearly all teenagers at one time or other.

PHYSICAL EXAMINATION

Acne occurs most frequently on the face, but can also occur on the back, chest, and upper arms. Four types of lesions are generally described. The mildest form is the common blackhead. This lesion results from plugged sebaceous glands. When these lesions are associated with inflammation, they are referred to as comedos. As the inflammatory process progresses, pustules and deep cystic lesions may develop. The latter two lesions generally are associated with significant infection and require aggressive management.

MANAGEMENT

Treatment of acne is directed at the underlying mechanisms responsible for the lesions. For the initial stage (blackheads), simple cleansing of the skin is effective. Washing two or three times a day with a mildly abrasive or antiseptic soap will usually suffice. Once comedos have developed, peeling agents, such as benzoyl peroxide should be added to the cleansing regimen. Pustular lesions warrant the use of topical and/or systemic antibiotics such as erythromycin or tetracycline. These should be used in addition to local measures. In the event that pustules do not respond or should cysts develop, the client should be referred to a dermatologist.

Educational efforts should emphasize a nutritious diet, adequate exercise, sparse use of oily cosmetics, and refraining from picking or squeezing lesions. In severe cases, adolescents may also need psychological support.

CASE STUDY

Annie is a 15-year-old brought in by her mother because of obesity. She states that her weight problem began at age 11. She attributes the weight problem to an inability to exercise, and to the eating habits of her family. Her mother is also overweight, but her father and two younger siblings are slender. She is grade-appropriate in the tenth grade and makes good marks (As and Bs). She describes her father and a younger sister as athletic but describes herself as poorly coordinated. She also dislikes gym and requests an excuse from gym class.

She admits to being teased about her weight and avoids some social situations because of this. The client has one close friend, has never dated, and is not sexually active. Annie admits to being jealous of her younger sister, and feels that her father shows the sister partiality because of her athletic ability. She also blames her mother for contributing to her obesity because she (her mother) is responsible for meals and is also overweight. The mother states that Annie has always been chubby, and that previous attempts to lose weight have met with little success. These efforts have been limited to elimination of certain types of "fattening" foods.

On physical examination, the client is 5' 4" tall and weighs 176 lbs. Her pulse is 72 and regular, and her blood pressure is 130/80. Head, eyes, ears, nose, and throat (HEENT) are unremarkable as is examination of the neck, heart, lungs, and abdomen. Secondary sexual development is stage IV, and she states that her menses began at age 12. The neurologic exam is normal and examination of the skin reveals blackheads and comedos on the face. Plotting the client's measurements on a growth curve reveals that she is greater than the 99% for weight and above the 75% for height. Diagnostic tests included a complete blood count, urinalysis, chemistry profile, and thyroid function test. All tests were normal. The latter test was performed because of a family history of thyroid disease.

MANAGEMENT PLAN

Initially, it was determined that Annie did want to lose weight. She was advised that only she could accomplish this task. At the onset, Annie was asked to determine the approximate number of calories she consumed in an average day. Based on her recall, this was estimated to be approximately 3600. Snack foods accounted for a large portion of these calories. These snacks were eaten primarily in the afternoon and evening while watching television or studying. She also recalled that she tended to eat after her father mentioned her weight to her, or talked of his or her sister's athletic accomplishments.

Annie was started on a 1200-calorie diet, and her mother's cooperation was enlisted to decrease the chances of snacking by making snack foods less available. Annie and her mother also joined a local health spa for regular planned exercise. They attended the spa every other day, and on alternate days they agreed to either walk or ride bikes for 30 to 60 minutes. Her father was asked to establish common interests with Annie and to build a positive relationship. It was suggested to him that Annie might not choose to participate in the sports activities that he and Annie's sister enjoyed.

Annie lost 20 lbs over the next six months while being seen an average of every two weeks. Subsequent reduction has been very slow, but she feels better about her appearance, her coordination and herself in general. Gym class is no longer a painful experience, and she has continued to attend classes at the health spa. She and her father appear to be relating better, and she has been able to get her mother to join her in her weight program.

DISCUSSION

A major goal in this case was to help Annie recognize the antecedents to her overeating. These included reactions to the nervous energy associated with watching TV and studying, and an urge to "get back at" her father for harassing her over her weight and inactivity. Family counseling also revealed that her mother and father had experienced long-term hostilities over the mother's sedentary life-style and obesity. Hopefully, Annie will be able to continue her weight loss through changed eating habits and increased physical activity.

STUDY QUESTIONS

Circle all that apply.

1. Obesity is a common problem during adolescence. Which of the following conditions is the most common underlying cause of obesity during adolescence?

a. hypothyroidism
b. diabetes mellitus
c. exogenous (overeating)
d. Cushing's syndrome

2. All but one of the following answers could be used to define obesity. Please indicate which answer is incorrect.

a. triceps skinfold thickness≥ 85th percentile
b. body weight in excess of 5% of calculated normal for age, height, and sex
c. body weight ≥ 90% of age, height, and weight
d. body weight greater than 10% of calculated normal for age, height, and sex

3. Although specific definitions for obesity are helpful, a majority of the time the diagnosis is evident to the clinician and client. A simple and useful indicator of an exogenous versus endocrine cause for obesity is the location of the client's height on a growth chart. Which one of the following clients is least likely to have exogenous obesity?

a. height 75%, weight > 99%
b. height 70%, weight > 99%
c. height 60%, weight > 99%
d. height 10%, weight > 99%

4. The basic mechanism for losing weight is to adjust caloric intake and expenditure. When caloric expenditure exceeds intake, weight loss will occur. Most clients will need assistance in accomplishing this task. Which of the following have proved useful in helping clients make needed adjustments?

a. joining a group
b. planning a diet
c. daily exercise
d. changing eating habits
e. all of above

5. Behavior modification is often helpful to individuals attempting to lose weight. The basics of this approach include all of the following except:

a. helping the client gain insight into eating habits
b. defining circumstances antecedent to eating
c. eating at least three meals a day
d. mastering control over eating

6. The case presented demonstrates the basic points of behavior modification. An early step is to identify antecedents to overeating. Annie was able to identify all of the following as either antecedents to overeating or associated with overeating, except one. Please indicate which one answer Annie was least likely to associate with overeating.

   a. pressure from her father
   b. comparing herself to her sister
   c. snacking while studying
   d. hunger

7. The client in this case study had acne on the face consisting of blackheads and comedos. Appropriate treatment would include all of the following except:

   a. cleansing twice daily
   b. topical steroid cream
   c. avoiding oily makeups
   d. topical benzoyl peroxide

ANSWERS

1. c   5. c
2. b   6. d
3. d   7. b
4. e

REFERENCES

1. Tanner, J. M. *Growth at adolescence*. (2nd Ed.). Oxford: Blackwell Scientific Publications Ltd., 1962.
2. The Alan Guttmacher Institute. *Adolescent pregnancy, the problem that hasn't gone away*. New York: Planned Parenthood Federation of America, 1980.
3. Friedman, F. B., & Sarles, R. M. "Out of control" behavior in adolescents. *Pediatric Clinics of North America*, 1980, *27*, 97.

BIBLIOGRAPHY

Baldwin, W. The children of teenage parents. *Family Panning Perspectives,* 1980, *12,* 34.

Felice, M. The young pregnant teenager: impact of comprehensive care. *Journal of Adolescent Health Care,* 1981, *1,* 193.

Friedman, F. B., & Sarles, R M, "Out of control" behavior in adolescents. *Pediatric Clinics of North America,* 1980, *27,* 97.

Gross, M. A. Treatment of obesity in adolescents using behavioral self-control. *Clinical Pediatrics,* 1976, *15,* 920.

Hatcher, R. A. *Contraceptive Technology, 1980–81.* New York: Irvington Publishers, 1980.

Heisler, A. B. Adolescence: psychological and social development. *Journal of School Health,* 1980, 381.

Marks, A. Aspects of biosocial screening and health maintenance in adolescents. *Pediatric Clinics of North America,* 1980, *27,* 153.

Parcel, G. Adolescent health concerns, problems and patterns of utilization in a triethnic urban population. *Pediatrics,* 1977, *60,* 157.

Rasmussen, J. E. A new look at old acne. *Pediatric Clinics of North America,* 1977, *25,* 285.

Smith, J. Interviewing adolescent patients: guidelines for the clinician. *Pediatric Annals,* 1980, *9,* 38.

Tanner, J. M. *Growth at adolescence.* 2nd ed. Oxford: Blackwell Scientific, 1962.

Adolescent pregnancy, the problem that hasn't gone away. New York: The Alan Guttmacher Institute, Planned Parenthood Federation of America 1980.

INDEX

Abdominal pain, 121–125
  in appendicitis, 121, 122
  in ascariasis, 139
  in colitis, 134
  diagnostic tests for, 126
  in inguinal hernia, 124
  in intussusception, 123
  management of, 126
  in mesenteric lymphadenitis, 124
  physical examination for, 126
  psychosomatic basis of, 125
  recurrent, 125–126
  from school phobia, 126
  in trichinosis, 140
Acne, 272
Adenoids, 170
Adolescence, 262–272
  acne during, 272
  alcohol and drug abuse during, 269–270
  behavior problems during, 268–269
  breast development in girls during, 262, 263
  developmental tasks in, 264
  diabetes mellitus in, 152
  enlargement of penis during, 263
  growth of pubic hair during, 263
  hormonal stimulation of gonadal function during, 262
  increased height in, 263
  obesity in, 270–272
  onset of menses during, 263
  puberty and, 262
  search for identity during, 263
  sexual activity during, 265–268
  testicular enlargement during, 263
  tinea cruris in, 201
Alcohol use, 269
Allergen:
  in allergic rhinitis, 52
  control of, in bronchial asthma, 59

  pollen, 53
  responses to, 53
Allergic disorder, 52
Allergic rhinitis:
  antigen-antibody interaction in, 53, 54
  causes of, 52
  conjunctivitis in, bilateral, 54
  diagnostic tests for, 54
  family counseling for, 55
  fatigue with, 53–54
  due to foods, 52
  histamine in, 53
  with increased susceptibility to colds, 54
  due to inhalants, 52, 53
  local inflammatory response in, 53
  management of, 55
    with antihistamines, 55–56
    with decongestants, 56
    with hyposensitization therapy (allergy shots), 56
  nasal smear for diagnosis of, 54–55
  perennial, 52
  periorbital edema in, 54
  physical examination for, 54
  runny nose in, 53
  seasonal, 52
  snoring due to, 53
  vasoactive enzymes in, 53
Allergic shiner, 53
American Academy of Pediatrics, 33
  preventive health care recommendations of, 34–35
    dental screening, 35
    development appraisal, 34
    measurements, 34
    physical examination, 35
    procedures, 35
    sensory screening, 34
  standards of, 34–35